Seeing Beauty,
Sensing Race
in Transnational Indonesia

Southeast Asia

POLITICS, MEANING, AND MEMORY
David Chandler and Rita Smith Kipp
SERIES EDITORS

Seeing Beauty, Sensing Race in Transnational Indonesia

L. AYU SARASWATI

University of Hawai'i Press
Honolulu

18   17   16   15   14   13   6   5   4   3   2   1

Library of Congress Cataloging-in-Publication Data
Saraswati, L. Ayu, author.
    Seeing beauty, sensing race in transnational Indonesia / L. Ayu Saraswati.
        pages cm. — (Southeast Asia—politics, meaning, and memory)
    Includes bibliographical references and index.
    ISBN 978-0-8248-3664-1 (cloth : alk. paper) — ISBN 978-0-8248-3736-5
(pbk. : alk. paper)
    1. Feminine beauty (Aesthetics)—Indonesia. 2. Human skin color—
Indonesia—Psychological aspects. 3. Race awareness—Indonesia. I. Title.
II. Series: Southeast Asia—politics, meaning, memory.
    HQ1220.I5S27 2013
    305.4209598—dc23
2012042310

University of Hawai'i Press books are printed on acid-free
paper and meet the guidelines for permanence and durability
of the Council on Library Resources.

Composition by Publishers' Design and Production Services, Inc.

Printed by Sheridan Books, Inc.

DEDICATED TO: DIZA, UTARI, AND CLAIRE

CONTENTS

ACKNOWLEDGMENTS

To all whose paths I have been lucky enough to cross: Thank you for teaching me how to gratefully embrace the sweetness of living and gracefully endure the challenges of life. All of you have been the strong anchors that lovingly and firmly hold my universe in its place.

Writing a scholarly book for over a decade must be a testament of one's love of knowledge and the arduous and fascinating process that goes along with it. I have been blessed with and am grateful for so many amazing souls whose love and commitment have also gone into the writing of this book. Claire Moses has, throughout more than a decade, provided me with constant and miraculous support in the making and remaking not only of this book but also of myself as a scholar, teacher, and person. I thank her for every victory, small and big, that I have been able to achieve, with her help of course, in my life.

I owe many thanks to the editors and anonymous reviewers at the University of Hawai'i Press for providing me with tremendously helpful feedback. This book is stronger because of them. I am grateful for Wendy Bolton's meticulous editing. Pamela Kelley has been an amazing editor to work with. She has made this process such an easy and wonderful one.

Professors and lifelong friends at the University of Maryland have unfailingly come to my rescue each time this book (or I) fell apart and needed restructuring. Seung-kyung Kim has been a firm and loving mentor; Debby Rosenfelt, Elsa Barkley Brown, Shawn Parry-Giles, Bonnie Thornton Dill, Lynn Bolles, Katie King, and Ruth Zambrana have all provided encouraging and inspiring space for me to grow intellectually, personally, and professionally. Annie Carter, Cliff Howard, and Laura Nichols have been there for me above and beyond their tremendous administrative help. Heather Rellihan, JV Sapinoso, Kim Willliams, Laura Logie, Robyn Epstein, and Gwyn Weathers have been such true, kind, and loving friends with whom I have enjoyed many stimulating conversations and some silly fun times. My thanks goes to each and every one of them.

Colleagues at Emory University provided me with a welcoming and intellectually stimulating home during my postdoc year there. Carla Freeman is a brilliant and encouraging scholar whose questions have made me rethink how I framed this book. Lynne Huffer, Pam Scully, Holloway Sparks, Rosemarie Garland-Thomson, and Esther Jones have all been wonderfully generous with their time and thought-provoking ideas. Berky Abreu and Linda Calloway tirelessly and patiently handled all administrative tasks. I thank them dearly.

It is to my colleagues at the University of Kansas whom I owe my learning to lead a balanced life: being productive while enjoying what life has to offer. Tanya Golash-Boza is an inspiring colleague whose solution-oriented approach to everything in life never allowed me a moment of unproductivity. Even when relaxing, I am "productive" in doing nothing! Incredibly loving and stimulating friendships with Mariya Omelicheva, Christina Lux, Tami Albin, Sherrie Tucker, Elif Andac, Randal Jelks, Stephanie Fitzgerald, Jessica Vasquez, Yajaira Padilla, Holly Thompson-Goerdel, Jorge Pérez, and Ben Chapell have all nurtured my development as a "soulful" scholar and person. My colleagues at the Department of Women, Gender, and Sexuality Studies at KU—Akiko Takeyama, Hannah Britton, Ann Schofield, Tanya Hart, Martha Vicente, Omofolabo Ajayi-Soyinka, John Younger, and Charlene Moehlenhard—have always been encouraging and nurturing every step of the way. Jan Emerson was very helpful with the incredible amount of administrative work I seemed to always have. The New Faculty General Research Fund, General Research Fund, and International Travel Research Grant of the University of Kansas have helped fund the research for this book. The Mary Savage Snouffer dissertation fellowship of the University of Maryland also contributed to the early writing of this book.

My colleagues in the Women's Studies Department at the University of Hawai'i—Mire Koikari, Kathy Ferguson, Meda Chesney-Lind, Susan Hippensteele, Aya Kimura, and Monisha Das Gupta—have all shared with me their brilliance, grace, encouragement, and positive energy. The magnitude of my gratitude for being able to work with them in this beautiful island simply goes beyond my ability to express it. I thank them for inviting me to be a part of their strong and vibrant department. Being here still often feels like a dream. I thoroughly enjoy taking intellectual delight in this poetic space of Hawai'i. Norine Young and Elliott Curelop have been wonderfully helpful with the administrative paperwork related to this book.

Throughout the years, I have also been blessed to have known these fantastic colleagues and friends scattered across the globe: Joanne Rondilla, Merlyna Lim, Pensri Ho, Abidin Kusno, Tineke Hellwig, Michael Bodden, Lila Kurnia, Arianne Nartyasari, Arnika Fuhrmann, and Manneke Budiman. They have all kindly shared their time and brilliant ideas with me as I've worked on this book. I sincerely and humbly thank them.

To the many women whose names remain anonymous, I thank them for sharing their stories and for trusting me to tell them. Thanks also to Dina and

Avi for letting me stay at their beautiful place by the beach during my research in the Netherlands.

My thanks also goes to the librarians at Perpustakaan Nasional Indonesia (The National Library of Indonesia) in Jakarta, and librarians and scholars, especially Rini Hogewoning and Dr. Henk Schulte Nordholt, at KITLV in Leiden and KIT in Amsterdam, the Netherlands. They have helped me locate and suggested many invaluable sources for my research.

My deepest gratitude also goes to my family. I thank my mother, Utari Koesumo, for never failing to keep me in her prayers, and for helping me get to where I am. She has enlightened and lightened whichever paths I have chosen to create for myself. My father, Sutji Prakoso, has helped me secure some materials that were much needed for this book. My sister, Agung Nugrahaeni, has always been incredibly generous and supportive and kindly accommodated my needs during my research stay in Indonesia and beyond. When I had to come up with an image for the cover, I first turned to one of the most talented and amazingly creative souls I admire and love dearly, my brother, Ibnu Magda. I thank him for his generosity with his time and brilliantly creative mind! Last but not least, thanks to Diza Edgina who has taught me to be immersed with love in whatever I am doing, being, and writing. This book is dedicated to her, with unwavering love.

An earlier version of chapter four appeared as "*Cosmopolitan Whiteness*: The Effects and Affects of Skin-Whitening Advertisements in Transnational Women's Magazine in Indonesia" in *Meridians* 10.2 (2010): 15–41. Earlier versions of parts of chapter five appeared as "*Malu*: Coloring Shame and Shaming the Color of Beauty in Transnational Indonesia" in *Feminist Studies* 38.1 (2012): 113–140.

Introduction

*Seeing Beauty, Sensing Race in
Transnational Indonesia*

In Indonesia, light skin has been the desirable color for as long as we can document. As this book will make clear, in some of the oldest surviving Indonesian literature, such as the epic poem *Ramayana*, adapted in the late ninth century from its Indian origin, light-skinned women were the dominant beauty norm of the time. In both the Indian and Indonesian versions of *Ramayana*, beautiful women are described as having white shining faces, like the full moon. One thousand years later during the early twentieth century when Dutch colonialism fully matured in Indonesia, images of Caucasian white beauty were used to illustrate the epitome of beauty in advertisements published in women's magazines. When Japan took over as the new colonial power in Indonesia from 1942 to 1945, they propagated a new *Asian* beauty ideal, but white remained the preferred skin color. In postcolonial Indonesia, particularly since the late 1960s when the pro-American president Soeharto reigned, American popular culture has become one of the strongest influences against which an Indonesian white beauty ideal is articulated and negotiated. These transnational circulations of beauty ideals throughout different historical periods have undoubtedly helped maintain the light-skinned preference and configure not only beauty, but also racial, gender, and skin color discourses in Indonesia. The popularity of skin-whitening products—ranked first among all revenue-generating products in the cosmetics industry in Indonesia—is further evidence of such light-skinned preference.

I will trace these circulations of beauty images from different countries to Indonesia from precolonial to postcolonial periods and explain how transnational circulations of beauty ideals help shape the construction of race, gender, and skin color in Indonesia. Moreover, I offer a fresh perspective on the transnational construction of categories of identity by telling this story through the lens of "affect" and emotion. By affect, I refer to philosopher Teresa Brennan's definition of the term as the "physiological shift accompanying a judgment" (2004, 5). It is how the body cringes at the sight of a feared subject or jolts as it catches a glimpse of a beautiful being. Understanding when, how, and why bodies feel certain affects toward specific bodies allows us to understand the larger social structures within which the meanings of these bodies and their responses make *sense*. In essence, this book is a theoretical exploration of the ways in which human emotions are made *visible* in and circulated through the representations of beauty images that travel across different geographical locations and how they help shape discourses and hierarchies of race, gender, and skin color transnationally.

Thus, I will pay careful and critical attention to how ideals of beauty that travel transnationally circulate "feelings" about people of specific race, skin color, and gender. It is through these feelings that meanings of race, gender, and skin color are registered. Anchoring my analysis in theories of affect and feminist cultural studies of emotions, I argue that race, gender, and skin color are affectively constructed. Pointing out the importance of feelings, senses, and affects in the processes of subjectivity formation in a transnational context, this book furthers our current understanding of race, gender, and skin color as visually and socially constructed.

SEEING AND SENSING

"Seeing is believing," the old saying goes. And even a postmodern philosopher such as Judith Butler who complicates the phrasing of the simple adage ("the visual field is not neutral to the question of race; it is itself a racial formation, an episteme, hegemonic and forceful") would agree on the importance of a visual field in our claim "to know" (1993, 17). According to both versions, the production of knowledge (and racial formation), or, perhaps, "truths," is inseparable from the structures within which our visual apparatus interprets the visual field, manipulated as it may be.

Scholars have argued that for people without visual impairments, vision is the most developed and most important faculty of all human senses; humans are visually oriented (Tuan 1974/1990, 6; Blauert 1983 quoted in Rodaway 1994, 92). Being seen, however, can be a double-edged sword. Although feminists operate under the premise that "being seen" is politically advantageous and desirable, race and feminist cultural studies scholars Sara Ahmed and Jackie Stacey caution that being seen may also lead to the unwanted effect of surveillance (Ahmed and Stacey 2000, 16).[1]

Like seeing, sensing is also an epistemic apparatus. Sensing provides us with the means through which we make sense of the "real" world and how to live in it (Rodaway 1994, 7; Davidson 2003, 92). Geographer Paul Rodaway defines senses[2] as:

> not merely passive receptors of particular kinds of environmental stimuli but . . . actively involved in the structuring of that information and . . . significant in the overall sense of a world achieved by the sentient. In this way, sense and reality are related. (1994, 4)

Thus, senses, as a critical apparatus in the process of knowledge production and subjectivity formation, "provid[e] us with both information about a world around us and, through their structure and the way we use them, . . . mediate that experience" (Rodaway 1994, 3). Because senses function as a tool of *knowing*, they are never innocent and are always historically, politically, and socially specific (Rodaway 1994, 7).

To rely on one's senses and render them useful in the process of knowledge production, however, is not to suggest that we cannot question their validity (Jaggar 1989, 163). Feminist philosopher Alison Jaggar pointed out, "emotions are not presocial, physiological responses to unequivocal situations, they are open to challenge on various grounds" (1989, 163). Thus, emotions are no more "authentic" than "reason" (Harding and Pribram 2009, 5–6). Nor can they function as a better "epistemological authority" in the process of knowledge production (Skeggs 2000, 28). Both emotion and reason are equally important and are inseparable from each other (Tuan 1977, 10; Jaggar 1989, 165). Indeed, going back to the ancient Indian tradition, feeling has been framed as something inseparable from thinking (Santoso 1980, 15). Incorporating emotions into our scholarship thus demands that we carve out "an epistemological basis" for their existence in our research (Harding and Pribram 2004, 882).

This book's examination of the circulations and representations of the human emotions in imagery representing beauty aims to reveal the ways in which power relations are articulated in gendered, racialized, colored, and transnationalized terms. The theoretical lens of affect helps us to do this because affect is articulated, circulated, and performed through relations of power (Harding and Pribram 2004, 17). Emotions can even function to obscure power relations and make them seem natural in everyday lives (Probyn quoted in Harding and Pribram 2009, 6). Considering affect as a system of power thus refers to the ways in which ideology of emotions regulates who can feel what, when, and how. Jaggar explains this clearly:

When unconventional emotional responses are experienced by isolated individuals, those concerned may be confused, unable to name their experience; they may even doubt their own sanity. Women may come to believe that they are "emotionally disturbed" and that the embarrassment or fear aroused in them by male sexual innuendo is prudery or paranoia. When certain emotions are shared or validated by others, however, the basis exists for forming a subculture defined by perceptions, norms, and values that systematically oppose the prevailing perceptions, norms, and values. By constituting the basis for such a subculture, outlaw emotions may be politically and epistemologically subversive. (1989, 160)

This book's attempt to map the gendered and racialized ideology of emotions represented in images of beauty thus speaks to its desire to chart how "power operates through affect" (Grossberg quoted in Harding and Pribram 2004, 872). By way of examining which signifiers are being used in which representations for which affective purposes, I intend to expose how affect functions as an apparatus of power that does the work of naturalizing various social hierarchies including racial, gender, and skin color hierarchies, in a transnational context. As such, I will make visible how power enters the domain of the emotions, or what Butler (1997a) called the "psychic life of power," and thus implicitly elucidates the ways in which we may be able to break free from the grip of power that enters, resides, and circulates within the sphere of emotions. In short, the book is an exploration of what anthropologist Catherine Lutz calls "emotion as an ideological practice" (1988, 4).

I emphasize the importance of sensing/feeling in the act of seeing. It is "see[ing] through an embodied, feeling engagement." The act of seeing is thus simultaneously an exercise of sensing because, as geographer Divya Tolia-Kelly pointed out, "we cannot 'see' and 'feel' separately; . . . aesthetics in representations are about emotions as much as they are about form, visual grammars permeate with visceral narrations of embodied values." That is, I frame feeling as not simply a "*context* to seeing" (Tolia-Kelly 2007, 340). Rather, feeling *is* a way of seeing the world.

WHY BEAUTY?

In this book, I render beauty an important subject of inquiry because it allows me to expose the simultaneous and intersecting ways in which racial, gender, skin color, transnational, and emotional/affective discourses work together in producing and maintaining power hierarchies. Hence, I employ beauty ideology as a critical lens to examine how whiteness, when viewed, articulated, and framed within the notion of female beauty, took on its gendered meanings. Certainly, in women's studies, the notion of beauty ideology as a discriminatory tool among women has been widely accepted. Some feminist scholars term discrimination against "ugly" women "look-ism" in order to expose the ways in which "beauty expectations are systemic" (Chancer 1998, 83). Some would even consider beauty or look-ism more dangerous than racism and sexism—the larger institutional structures upon which it hinges—because we are aware of discrimination based on race and sex, we are rather unaware or "unconscious" about discrimination based on looks (Etcoff 1999, 25). Beauty ideology has indeed been used to keep modern women in their subordinate place (Wolf 1992). This is because the never-ending beauty rituals, in Foucauldian terms, "discipline" women's bodies differently from men's and even manufacture them as "docile bodies" (Bartky 1990, 69–75).

Scholars suggest that beauty becomes a discriminatory tool because of its capital form. Sociologist Lynn Chancer, in working with Pierre Bordieu's notion of "cultural capital," argues that beauty can be *worked at* and *worked for*: looks are not merely ascribed but more and more frequently *achieved*" (1998, 118). Women are therefore invested in working at and for beauty because, as a form of capital, beauty is "transformable into other types of capital, such as economic capital or money. The amount of beauty a woman possesses may help her land a well-paying job or marry a high-status, wealthy man" (M. Hunter 2005, 5).

Of particular interest for me is the increasingly popular use of skin-whitening creams, particularly in Indonesia. Historically, it must be noted, skin-whitening products were not limited to African or Asian peoples; nor are they a recent invention of capitalism and the global cosmetics industry. From race scholar Richard Dyer's research, we learn that women in ancient Greece were already concerned with whitening their skin (1997, 48). Women during the Roman Empire used ceruse and white lead to whiten their skin. In Elizabethan England (sixteenth to early seventeenth century), ceruse was used for the same purpose (Sherrow 2001, 241). Some other ingredients used were mercury, lemon juice, egg whites, milk, and vinegar (Etcoff 1999, 101). Indeed, because ingredients such as lead and mercury are poisonous, women have died because of these practices (Sherrow 2001, 86).

In the North American context, women have also practiced whitening routines. Historian Kathy Peiss noted that during the early nineteenth century, white women were sharing recipes for skin whiteners and until the twentieth century were the target market for bleaching creams. In the mid-nineteenth century, the press began to notice the use of skin whiteners among African Americans (Peiss 1998, 9, 41, 149). Until the early twentieth century, African Americans continued to be targeted for whitening products with damaging chemicals, including mercury, which was banned in the United States only in 1974 (Sherrow 2001, 242).

In Asia and Africa, whitening practices have also been historically popular. The Egyptian queen Cleopatra would take milk baths to whiten her skin (Dyer 1997, 48; Sherrow 2001, 35). In the ninth to twelfth centuries, Japan's Heian period, women used rice flour (oshiroi) and white lead to whiten their skin (Etcoff 1999, 101). In thirteenth-century China, rich women would use "Buddha's adornment"—thick paste applied to their face during the winter that they removed in spring (Sherrow 2001, 76). In modern Zimbabwe, skin whiteners were used until they were banned in 1980 (Burke 1996, 120).

These examples of whitening practices that have existed in various geographical locations and historical periods provide the context for rethinking the issue of beauty and skin color in a transnational context. That women in various nations, including Indonesia and the United States, have admitted to desiring light skin so that they can look "beautiful"; and the fact that skin-whitening products are popular in many nations, such as Zimbabwe, Nigeria, Ivory Coast, the Gambia, Tanzania, Senegal, Mali, Togo, Ghana, Vietnam, Malawi, Philippines, Singapore, Malaysia, Japan, China, Saudi Arabia (and the list goes on), provides overwhelming evidence that a beauty discourse that privileges light-skinned women circulates transnationally. Indeed, thinking transnationally is not only important but also inevitable. The materials gathered in this book came from three countries: the United States, from the Library of Congress in Washington, D.C.; Indonesia, from Arsip Nasional Republik Indonesia (the National Archive of the Republic of Indonesia), and Perpustakaan Nasional Indonesia (the National Library of Indonesia) in Jakarta; and the Netherlands, from the KITLV library in Leiden and KIT library in Amsterdam.

In proposing and employing a different way of seeing beauty—one that relies on, makes visible, and is facilitated by feelings—this book produces different knowledges, histories, and understandings about beauty, racial, gender, and skin color discourses, particularly in Indonesia. That is, I reframe the complexity of beauty practices as neither victimizing nor empowering but rather as a mode of feeling and managing these feelings in a transnational context.

WHY INDONESIA?

Does the widespread use of skin-whitening cosmetic products point to a universal experience of race, and/or gendered race? Scholars have questioned this, pointing instead to the local histories in which race is constructed. As race scholars Perry Hintzen and Jean Rahier have written, although in the United States subjectivity is deeply racialized, "perhaps, in other national spaces, race is overwhelmed by other ways of knowing, other discourses of being, other subjectivities" (2003, 15). This suggests that scholars who are interested in race, racial formation, and racialization and have focused on the American model may not fully conceptualize race in other places and in a transnational context. Focusing on Indonesia whose history is very different from that of the United States thus allows me to expand our understanding of and offer a different knowledge about how race, gender, and color are constructed. Moreover, Indonesia would seem to be an excellent example for proving their suspicion: the specificity of Indonesian racial history, racial (un)consciousness and racial make-up, and the fact that most people in contemporary Indonesia do not think through the lens of race, are often used to dismiss attempts to discuss race and color issues there. Although this book takes issue with that stance by insisting on the importance of racially signified skin color in Indonesia, the book does show the multiple ways in which the construction of racially signified skin color in Indonesia is different from the "lighter-the-better" construction of skin color so prevalent in the U.S. context. For example, in chapter five, I discuss the Indonesian approval of a so-called Japanese white skin color but disdain for "Chinese" white skin color. Moreover, other categories of identity such as gender, also matter in our understanding the meanings of skin color. Thus, while women are expected to care for their skin color and are considered beautiful when their skin is light, men are not. In Indonesia, light skin color is associated with femininity. Nonetheless, it would be a mistake to view Indonesia as a closed society with only local or national explanations for its gender and racial attitudes. Framing the issue of beauty in a transnational context allows me to identify the specificity of race in Indonesia with a specificity that is transnational.

Indonesia, located in the southeast of Asia with neighboring countries such as Malaysia, Singapore, Brunei, East Timor, New Guinea, and Australia, is a modern and postcolonial invention. It was established as a nation-state only after its independence in 1945. Prior to that, it was colonized by the Dutch who ruled over various kingdoms, scattered throughout this vast archipelago that consists of 17,508 islands (6,000 inhabited). Hence, the geographical boundaries of today's Indonesia are mostly a legacy of Dutch colonialism. Dutch colonialism also helps explain, as Southeast Asian specialist Benedict Anderson pointed out, why Indonesians of Sumatran ethnicity would consider Malaysia's Malays, with whom they share language, religion, and ethnicity, "foreigners," yet consider the Ambonese in Eastern Indonesia, with whom they share no such commonalities, as fellow Indonesians, belonging to the same "imagined community." This is so simply because they were colonized by the same colonizer (Anderson 1983/2006, 120–121). Even Indonesia's insistence on "integrating" Irian or West Papua into Indonesia was due partly to the fact that Irian was once a Dutch colony and thus became part of the Indonesian imaginary. In contrast, East Timor, an island that was once colonized by the Portuguese but was then "occupied" by Indonesia in 1975, is now an independent country.

Even the word itself, Indonesia, is a European invention. It was only in 1850, in the *Journal of the Indian Archipelago and Eastern Asia*, that its co-editor, James Richardson Logan, created the name "Indonesia," selecting from one of the two names—"Indunesia" (Indian archipelago) and "Malayunesia" (Malay archipelago)—that his co-editor, George Samuel Windsor Earl, had proposed in an earlier article in the same journal (Anshory 2004). Logan chose Indunesia but changed the letter *u* to *o* to make it sound better. Then, because he persistently used the word Indonesia in his publications, the word became more and more popular. In 1884, Djerman Bastian used "Indonesia" to title a book he wrote about the archipelago (Stoddard 1966, 278). And by 1913, when one of Indonesia's twentieth-century nationalist heroes and founder of *Indonesische Persbureau*, Ki Hajar Dewantara, began to use the word "Indonesia" in his newspaper to refer to this geographical location, it was evident that the name had taken hold (Anshory 2004).

The national language of Indonesia is Indonesian (*Bahasa Indonesia*).[3] It has been acknowledged as the national language since 1928; however, it was only in 1942 with the beginning of Japanese occupation that Indonesian achieved the "de facto status of official language"; and in 1945, following the country's independence, Indonesian officially became the country's national language (Sneddon 2003, 9). Indonesian is a language that was derived from "high" or "formal" Malay.[4] The "low" form of Malay[5] was spoken, at least until the early twentieth century, alongside approximately 550 dialects including the most-widely spoken dialect, Javanese, and Chinese (Sneddon 2003, 5). Certainly, circulations of people and objects from various places influenced the rich and shifting languages spoken in Indonesia. For example, the Old Javanese language, or *Kawi* (written prior to the fifteenth century), was a dominant language among the Javanese literati and people of the royal courts prior to European colonization (Phalgunadi 1995, 5). The Dutch[6] and Portuguese then brought their languages to the archipelago in the sixteenth century adding to the variety of languages already spoken.

Indonesia is a big country both in terms of its size (crossing three time zones)[7] and its population (it is the largest Muslim country and the fourth most populous country in the world with an estimated 238 million people in 2010). Some theorists suggest that the "original" inhabitants of Indonesia, possibly about 30,000–40,000 years ago, were dark-skinned people (Vlekke 1960, 8; Mirpuri 1990, 19), and that migrations of people from various locations to the archipelago have contributed to the mixture of people in today's Indonesia (Mirpuri 1990,

54). Historian Jean Gelman Taylor, however, suggests that differences that exist in today's Indonesia are not a result of migrations by different races of people, but rather they reflect the different ways in which people adapted to changes brought about by transnationally circulated objects and people; she argues that the predecessors of most of today's Indonesians came from Southern China (J. Taylor 2003, 5–7).

Nonetheless, Indonesia has a long history of transnational circulations of people that continues to the present day. Encounters with Indians, Chinese, and Arabs during the precolonial period; the experience of Dutch colonialism that differs significantly from English and French colonial models; and the experience of Japanese colonialism and encounters with American culture in the contemporary period make Indonesia unique and an important site of analysis. Based on 2004 data, foreign workers (not necessarily Caucasian) in Indonesia number about 20,000 (6,000 executives, 11,600 professionals, 1,200 supervisors, 500 technicians, and the rest, "other").[8] More than half of these workers live in Jakarta.

This examination of the construction of race, gender, and skin color in Indonesia stands on the shoulders of prominent scholarship on race and gender in Indonesia (Stoler 2002; Gouda 1995; Hellwig 1994; Locher-Scholten 1986, 1992, 2000; Foulcher and Day 2002). However, these studies on race and gender in Indonesia have tended to focus on colonial and postcolonial periods. In contrast, I broaden the focus by examining the transnational history of skin color, racial, and gender formation in Indonesia in the precolonial period and then trace these formations through to the present day.

STRUCTURE OF THE BOOK

This book has as its anchors the field of feminist cultural studies of emotions and affect theories. Each chapter offers theoretical frameworks that build on and enrich existing theories on senses, feelings, emotions, and affects. I need to clarify here that I use the notion of "senses" as a theoretical placeholder to which I hook other theoretical concepts related to "sensing," such as affects, feelings, emotions, and "sensing" concepts specific to Indonesia and South/Southeast Asia such as *rasa* and *malu*. Hence, I interweave, work with, and build on these concepts at different moments, creating a tapestry of theories of emotions in the process. Simultaneously, these theoretical concepts help explain and move forward the historically specific narratives told in every chapter.

In chapter one, "*Rasa*, Race, and *Ramayana*: Sensing and Censoring the History of Color in Precolonial Java," I introduce the theoretical concept of *rasa* and deploy it to construct a historical account of skin color and gender hierarchies in late-ninth-century and early-tenth-century Java, prior to European colonization. The choice to begin my story with a precolonial period reflects my attempt to refrain from (re)producing a "Eurocentric" text in which the beginning of history is marked by (encounters with) Western/colonial history (Shohat and Stam 1994). Unfortunately, materials from and about this particular period are scarce. There are, however, a limited number of precolonial Old Javanese-language *kakawin* (poems) that have been translated into modern Indonesian and English. To this end, I chose to analyze one of the most popular epic stories from that period, *Ramayana*.

Through a reading of the Old Javanese adaptation of the Indian epic poem *Ramayana*, chapter one argues that color hierarchy already mattered prior to European colonialism and was articulated through affective vocabularies attached to notions of beauty. The chapter argues that the conflation between lightness and light skin as desirable and darkness and dark skin as undesirable is registered through *rasa*. That is, in *Ramayana*, women with light skin color are represented with positive *rasa* as beautiful and desirable, whereas people with dark skin color are represented with negative *rasa* as undesirable and often terrifying.

I define *rasa* as a dominant emotion found when encountering (and in) performative events and characters that provoke our "affective trajectories" and previously "deposited memory elements" (Higgins 2007, 47). I distinguish *rasa* from its theoretical affiliations of affect and emotion in that, while affect is understood as bodily reactions to certain experiences, and emotion is the social expression of that affect, *rasa* is the emotion that underlies and is attached to a performative event/representation. *Rasa* can be found in the text itself as well as felt by the audience reading the text/performance/representation.

In chapter two, "Rooting and Routing Whiteness in Colonial Indonesia: From Dutch to Japanese Whiteness," I work with the concept of emotion and develop this further as "colonial emotionology." Emotion,[9] unlike affect, registers at the level of the social interpretation of these bodily shifts (Conradson and Latham 2007, 236). Thus the expressions of emotions are usually, except for facial and tonal expressions that are deemed more universal, culturally specific (Thrift 2008, 181). In this sense, emotions are ideologically mediated (Harding and Pribram 2004, 875).

Because expressions of emotions are filtered through ideology, I develop a theoretical concept I call "colonial emotionology" to help us understand the ways in which subjectivity formation functions as an effect of ideology of emotions. Attaching notions of emotions to ideology certainly bespeaks and reveals the ways in which emotions function as an apparatus of power that does the work of naturalizing social hierarchies. Particularly, I focus on the construction of two categories of whiteness during two colonial periods: Dutch and Japanese whiteness. (The third and fourth categories of whiteness, Indonesian whiteness and

Cosmopolitan whiteness, are discussed in chapters three and four respectively.) I define "colonial emotionology" as the ways in which ideologically permitted emotions as an articulation of the self serve the interests of the colonial empire.

Moreover, in this chapter I further argue that the conflation between race and skin color in colonial Indonesia was affectively rooted in Dutch colonialism (1900–1942). The Japanese colonizer (1942–1945) then challenged and rerouted this conflation. Japanese people propagated their version of white beauty that is rooted not in their white race but in their white skin color. The argument is based on historical and discursive analyses of beauty advertisements published in women's magazines such as *De Huisvrouw* (1938–1939), *De Huisvrouw in Deli* (1933–1935), *De Huisvrouw in Indie* (1933, 1936, 1937, 1940–1941), *De Huisvrouw in Nord Sumatra* (1939–1940), and *Vereniging van Huisvrouwen Cheribon* (1936); Japanese propaganda periodicals, such as *Djawa Baroe* (1943–1945) and *Almanak Asia Raya* (1943); and the "native," Chinese, and Arab periodicals *Bintang Hindia* (1928), *Fu Len* (1938), *Keng Po* (1933, 1938), *Pewarta Arab* (1933), and *Soeara Asia* (1943–1944).

Moving beyond the colonial periods of Indonesian history, chapter three, "Indonesian White Beauty: Spatializing Race and Racializing Spatial Tropes," develops a concept of emotionscape. This takes us to the second half of twentieth-century Indonesia during the post-Independence era under Soekarno until the end of Indonesia's second president Soeharto's regime in 1998. Here, our focus shifts to the importance of space, particularly during the nation-building period, and shows how various spatial tropes and the affective meanings they signify were visually deployed in advertisements to construct the racialized self and other. That is, I argue that the nationalized geographical space of Indonesia became a useful signifier to provide meanings for an "Indonesian" white beauty category. The deployment of such spatial tropes is implicit in and relies on the transnational production of affects about these places and the racial categories that are signified by them. Moreover, in highlighting the importance of spatial tropes that provide meanings for race and skin color, this chapter provides evidence for the construction of a category of whiteness I call "Indonesian white." This construction reshapes the relationship among concepts of gender, race, skin color, space, and nation.

This attachment between space, race, and emotions is articulated through the theoretical concept of emotionscape. Emotionscape helps us understand better the ways in which emotions travel and circulate transnationally and form a landscape—a repertoire and a repository—of dominant feelings about certain objects (i.e., race, place, skin color, white beauty) to which these emotions (i.e., fear, happiness, love) are attached. I define emotionscape as a repository of culturally scripted and socially acceptable emotions that circulate transnationally throughout different historical periods. Simultaneously, emotionscape is a repertoire of possible emotions from which people draw when they produce and reproduce representations, images, and narratives about and attach emotional meanings to certain objects. Examples that help explain this concept and provide evidence for the construction of Indonesian whiteness derive from discourse and historical analyses of beauty ads published in *De Huisvrouw in Indonesie* (1949), *De Huisvrouw* (1951, 1954, 1955, 1956), *Dunia Wanita* (1952, 1956, 1957), *Ketjantikan* (1953), *Wanita* (1949–1953, 1956–1957), *Pantjawarna* (1948, 1957, 1958, 1959), *Puspa Wanita* (1958, 1960), *Suara Perwari* (1951, 1953–1955, 1957–1958), *Warta* (1959–1960), and *Femina* (1975–1998).

In chapter four, "*Cosmopolitan* Whiteness: The Effects and Affects of Skin-Whitening Advertisements in a Transnational Women's Magazine," I employ discourse and semiotic analyses (Leiss et al. 1986, 150) to decode the meanings of various "signs" in whitening advertisements published in the Indonesian edition of *Cosmopolitan* magazine and tanning advertisements in the American *Cosmopolitan* during the years 2006 to 2008. Here, I challenge the assumption that "white" can only mean Caucasian white. I argue that it is "Cosmopolitan whiteness" (a category of whiteness that is different from, yet may include, Caucasian whiteness) that is being marketed through these whitening ads. Whiteness is not simply racialized or nationalized as such, but transnationalized. It is represented as, or equated with, "cosmopolitanness," embodying transnational mobility and transcending race and nation. In this chapter, I also argue that gender, race, and skin color are "affectively" constructed.

Hence, if in chapters two and three I rely on beauty ads to chart the historical shift of white beauty ideals during two colonial periods and the post-Independence era, in chapter four, I "read" these advertisements as "texts" using a discourse analysis to uncover their operating racial, gender, and skin color discourses. Moreover, I also add another layer of analysis by employing theories of affect and cultural studies of emotions. Thus, I decode not only the meanings of these images, but also the emotions represented by the gendered and racialized models in these ads.

In chapter five, "*Malu*: Coloring Shame and Shaming the Color of Beauty," I use the concept of *malu* (Indonesian word for shyness, embarrassment, shame, or restraint and propriety) as a lens through which I make sense of my interviews with forty-six Indonesian women and to argue that women's decision to practice (or not practice) skin-whitening routines is shaped by what I call "the gendered management of affect." The theoretical genealogy of "gendered management of affect" can be found in theories that frame affects, emotions, and feelings as a disciplinary technique: how we feel matters because this shapes how and what we do about our feelings (Harding and Pribram 2002; Ahmed 2004a, 2010). This chapter illustrates the gendered ways in which emotions and affects are managed and argues that performing beauty practices such as whitening one's skin is a manifestation of the gendered management of affects. Specifically, whitening practices reveal the gendered ways in which the feeling of *malu* is managed. Thus, chapter five points to the centrality of emotions in women's experiencing and negotiating discourses of beauty, race, skin color, and gender in their daily lives. These interviews reveal how affects and emotions function to naturalize difference and social hierarchies in a transnational context.

I end with a conclusion that pulls the chapters together to provide the theoretical implications of the book. By making affective production visible in the process of racial formation and showing the ways in which the meanings of race are registered through affect/emotion/feeling/*rasa/malu*, this book reworks the notion of race and suggests how race could be useful as an analytical category in a transnational context. That is, focusing on subjectivity formation as an effect of ideology of emotions affords me the possibility to show that by anchoring my analysis on affect theories, I am able to productively use the analytical category of race in a transnational context and in the process rethink the notion of "race," i.e., as affectively constructed. Certainly, this move toward "affect" studies is important particularly because key studies that highlight the ideological work and material consequences of race (Omi and Winant 1994; Winant 1994, 2001; Dyer 1997; M. Hunter 2005) have overlooked the ways in which feelings contribute to and are central in the gendered processes of racialization and subjectivity formation in a transnational context.

As a whole, this book adds to existing literatures on globalization by pointing out the importance of emotions in narratives of globalization. That is, although there has been much written on how people and objects that travel across national boundaries help transform the physical, cultural, social, racial, political, and financial landscape of the places they have traveled to and from (Appadurai1996; Lowe 1996; Ong 1999; Sarker and Niyogi De, 2002; Shohat 1998), little attention has been given to how circulations of people and ideas across national boundaries influence "the gendered management of affects": how people manage their feelings along gendered lines. The few exceptions that have begun to chart emotions in global context do not focus on Indonesia (Grewal 2005; Harding and Pribram 2009) or on racialized beauty (Wieringa 2007; Lindquist 2009).

In some ways, this book indeed attempts to paint a different picture of globalization. This book represents globalization as a narrative that is deeply embedded in the ebbs and flows of the formation of the nation rather than as "one-way" (cultural imperialism by the West) or "two-way" directions of power (both the West and the East influencing each other). Indonesia has never been an idyllic place to begin with. Even prior to the European conquest, transnational circulations of people, ideas, and images from different parts of the world, such as India, have all colored, quite literally, the cultural and physical landscape of Indonesia. Indonesia has indeed been a constantly changing place that keeps reconfiguring itself, and globalization is certainly one of the dominant narratives that could help explain these changes.

It certainly is possible to read the chapters in this book in whichever order serves one's needs best. Each chapter is indeed meant to stand on its own: it is written to represent distinct historical periods, countries, and sites of analysis. The specific sites and historical periods that are discussed in this book are meant to provide fragmentary snippets of societies that would become, are, and continue to be parts of Indonesian society at different moments in history. However, this book may best be read linearly: the chapters are organized to build on each other conceptually and, in some ways, to provide a sense of historical time. Each chapter focuses on different theoretical modalities of affect/feeling/emotion/sense/*rasa*/*malu* and each further strengthens my argument that race, color, and gender are affectively constructed in a transnational context. In whichever way this book is read, I hope it can serve its purpose as an exercise to theoretically mine the representations of human emotions with an open mind.

1 | *Rasa*, Race, and *Ramayana*

Sensing and Censoring the History of Color in Precolonial Java

History *affects* us. Historical narratives of colonialism and slavery may provoke our anger; tales of freedom and independence can awaken our courage and hope. One may wonder, however, if and how *affect* affects history. Indeed, when we make visible the underlying emotions that linger in history and shape how history is constructed, how and *will* the past be understood differently? My intention is to document the ways in which the circulations of an ideal beauty helped shape discourses of gender, skin color, and "race" during the late ninth and early tenth century in pre-European colonial Java, specifically in the Old Javanese adaptation of the Indian epic poem *Ramayana*. Focusing on the circulation of beauty ideals from India is important because India was the most prominent influence in the Indonesian archipelago prior to the establishment of Islamic kingdoms and European colonialism. The documentation of this circulation of beauty ideals will demonstrate how our understanding of precolonial and transnational histories of skin color, as they intersect with gender, shift when we employ a theoretical lens of affect and emotion in reading and constructing such histories.

As a re-telling of precolonial history that is sensitive to the ways in which emotion shapes history, this chapter argues that skin color already mattered prior to European colonialism and was articulated through affective vocabularies attached to notions of beauty. This argument challenges existing works that view colorism as rooted in European colonialism (Burke 1996; Sahay and Piran 1997; M. Hunter 2005). Arguing that preference for light skin color in Java predates European colonialism is not to argue that the construction of women with light skin color as beautiful is a "local" or "indigenous" construction (to be pitted against a "globalized" or Westernized construction) and that it has forever existed in indigenous communities, even without the force of European colonialism. Nor does it suggest that preference for light skin color is inherent in humanity. Far from it. The idea that it is light skin color that is considered beautiful, even in precolonial Java, I argue, is a "transnational" (*avant la lettre*) construction.[1]

Because I argue that meanings of skin color are constructed transnationally, it only makes sense that the lens through which I examine this issue is also a transnational one. To this end, I employ a "transnational" theoretical concept called *rasa*, which is rooted in precolonial Indian society and adapted to the Javanese context. In its Indian context, *rasa* is a theory most often used in regard to the audience's responses to works of performing art. In the Javanese context, *rasa* can be loosely translated as "the underlying emotion or mood which defines a work of art" (Saran and Khanna 2004, 12). *Rasa* is also registered in the Javanese spiritual world as a useful concept that could help explain how knowledge is produced both through senses and by sensing the unseen. I develop *rasa* fully cognizant of its transnational routes and meanings—these meanings include "mood," "emotional tone," "sentiment," or "feeling" (Higgins 2007, 45; Walton 2007, 31). I define *rasa* as a dominant emotion felt when encountering performative events and characters that provoke what philosopher Kathleen Higgins calls "affective trajectories" and previously "deposited memory elements" (47).

By developing and employing *rasa*, I provide evidence for how we can offer a different history of skin color and gender in precolonial Java when we pay attention to the emotions that curl languidly behind the stories we are reading. Hence I find it useful to provide specific examples of (1) how *rasa* functions as an apparatus through which we can sense skin color hierarchies within beauty discourse in precolonial Java and (2) how *rasa* functions as an apparatus of censorship in the production of a history of color in the Indonesian context. I do so by affectively reading the transnational epic poem *Ramayana*.

RAMAYANA: LITERARY TEXT AS HISTORICAL SOURCE

For this chapter, I focus mostly on the island of Java recognizing that there are more than 17,000 islands in Indonesia. I do so because Java has been one of the most developed and populated islands in the archipelago. During the Dutch colonial period, Java's economy became unquestionably the most developed; in contrast, in some other parts of Indonesia, especially eastern Indonesia, the economy can best be described as a "vacuum" (Dick 1996, 24). Today, the distribution of Indonesian people throughout its thousands of islands continues to be unevenly balanced. More than half of the population, about 130 million people, live on the island of Java. The rest are spread out across Sumatra (46 million), Sulawesi (15 million), and Kalimantan (12 million); only 16 million live on the other (approximately 6,000) inhabited islands. Java-centric politics continues to the present day, even after a policy of decentralization, implemented in 1999, began to gradually empower the other islands.

There is an extensive scholarship on early Indonesia. Much of it focuses on or begins with Java. The importance of Java and Javanese myths and culture cannot be overestimated because even in today's Indonesia, Javanese culture continues to be one of the most dominant in Indonesia and (mis)appropriated to serve the interests of the Javanese ruling elites. Javanese epics and myths are evoked to maintain the status quo in modern Indonesia (Hellwig 1994, 95; Tong 1999, 483).

As I mentioned in the introduction, Indonesia became a nation-state only after independence. Prior to that, several kingdoms ruled this vast archipelago. Indonesia's history records that at least by 400 CE there existed the kingdoms of Tarumanegara (West Java) and Kutai (East Kalimantan). The people in this archipelago had been immersed in circulations of people as parts of the trading market, even possibly since 2000 BCE, although it wasn't until the fifth century that the archipelago was squarely and strategically located as part of the larger trade network that included China and India (Drakeley 2005, 9, 10–11).

Royal inscriptions on stones, the earliest "written" documentations in the archipelago, have been useful for historians to construct a narrative of the past although they do not provide comprehensive information about the complex structures of their social, political, and economic lives (Creese 2004, 33–34). We simply know, based on these inscriptions, that people in Java at the time came from many different classes and held various occupations (J. Taylor 2003, 33). During this time, the royal kings controlled their people by giving their subordinates regional rulers autonomy and wealth in exchange for support; constructing a supernatural myth to explain their power; and having a strong army (Ricklefs 2008/2001, 19). These royal families also liked to build temples to honor Hindu gods and the Buddha (J. Taylor 2003, 35). Buddhism began to have significant presence in Java around 423 CE (Chatterji 1967, 7).

The earliest writing system in the archipelago was south Indian Pallawa script (Chatterji 1967, 5–6). In the course of centuries, it evolved into *Kawi* or the Old Javanese language (Drakeley 2005, 16). This is the language used in the original epic poem I will discuss. These Old Javanese narrative poems are called *kakawins*. They were written between the ninth and sixteenth centuries by male court poets for their kings (J. Taylor 2003, 32; Creese 2004, 38). They are usually hundreds of stanzas in length and were written based on "a set number of syllables per line, in fixed patterns of long and short syllables," following its Sanskrit literature origin (Creese 2004, 7). Although *kakawins* were mainly produced to pay homage to the kings and were often commissioned by these kings, they were composed to be performed through singing, dancing, playacting, and "clowning" in public spaces for people of different walks of lives (Creese 2004, 23; K. Hall 2005, 4). These *kakawins* have as their goals the maintenance of spiritual well-being of all who hear them (Creese 2004, 20).

If Indonesia did not exist prior to its formation in modern times, then what do we know about Indonesia prior to European colonization? Secondary sources tell us that one of the most dominant influences in precolonial Indonesia was India. Indeed, circulations of people and ideas from India reshaped the cultural terrain of the archipelago. This influence, according to some scholars, may have existed since the first century CE or perhaps even earlier, although its prominent influence can be observed only from the ninth century (Coedès 1968, 18–19; H. Sarkar 1970, 2–3, 20; Djamaris 1984, 16). An Indian legacy of sculptures and scriptures, produced during the first millennium and found throughout Southeast Asia, provides evidence for India's influence in this region (Walton 2007, 32). In Java, tangible legacies such as the *candi* (temples) of Prambanan and Borobudur function as physical testimonies to the ways in which Indian culture shaped, quite literally, the cultural landscape of precolonial Java (Hellwig and Tagliacozzo 2009, 14). In addition to these tangible legacies, intangible legacies such as values and religious systems also provide evidence for how India imprinted its culture on Java and its form of government. For example, contacts with India influenced the creation of caste in Java and Bali (Mulyana 1979, 199; Creese 2004, 117). This caste system, particularly during the Majapahit era (thirteenth to sixteenth centuries) in Java, might have incorporated race as a marker of distinction. For example, the three lowest groups who were excluded from society, as written in Negarakertagama LXXXI/4, were *candala* ("mixed" status/ race), *mleccha* (non-Aryan), and *tuccha* (useless people or criminals—*penjahat*) (Mulyana 1979, 206–207). And although the race/ethnicity of the Brahman and Ksatriya castes is uncertain (possibly Indian or Indianized Javanese), it has been argued that the Waisya or the merchant caste, at least in precolonial Bali, were people of Chinese, Mandar, and Bugis descent (Dwipayana 2001, 110).

Various reasons, from the technological (the development of passengerships) to the cultural (the development of Buddhism) to the commercial (trade in gold and spices), may have led Indians to the archipelago (Coedès 1968, 20–21; H. Sarkar 1970, 4–5). It is generally thought that merchants and traders in gold and spices were the first to develop ongoing contact with the islands; however, it was contact with north Indian Brahmins, the priestly caste, and in some cases with Ksatriya, the political ruling caste, rather than the Waisya, the merchant caste, or the lowest-caste Sudras, that brought Indian culture to Indonesia (Vlekke 1960, 24–25; Coedès 1968, 23; H. Sarkar 1970, 21, 27; Phalgunadi 1995, 1–2; J. Taylor

2003, 44–45; Dhoraisingam 2006). It was Brahmins, for example, who brought ideas about kingship to Java and then occupied positions not only as priests but also as "court poets, ministers of state, scribes, and record keepers" (Asher and Talbot 2006, 13). Scholars who argue that the Indian influence in Indonesia is a result of "Brahmanization" rather than large-scale migration from India point out that written evidence of Indian influence, particularly from the tenth century, is in Sanskrit. They argue that because this language is an elite and not a common language in India, it would have been impossible for commoners such as Indian merchants to have brought this language to Indonesia (Coedès 1968, 11–15; Zoetmulder 1974, 8–9).

In addition to contact with Brahmins, contact with the ruling elite, men of the Indian Ksatriya caste, also contributed to the Indianization of the archipelago. Kings, at least since the third century CE, bear Sanskrit names and are said to have some Indian origin or at least were Indianized (Coedès 1968, 25, 36). Indeed, these kings may have been Indians who migrated to the archipelago and founded their own small kingdoms. In other cases they may have been natives who became "Indianized" by visiting India, adopting Indian culture, or marrying an Indian princess to justify their rule (Coedès 1968, 24; H. Sarkar 1970, 36; Phalgunadi 1995, 1–2). Kings would sometimes also send their ambassadors to India, who would then bring back Indian ideas and practices, complementing (however partially) the process of Indianization in the archipelago (Vlekke 1960, 24).

Indianization was not a mere process of copying Indian culture, of course. During the precolonial period Javanese people carefully selected and adapted certain aspects of Indian culture to enrich their own cultural repertoires. As Indonesian studies scholars Tineke Hellwig and Eric Tagliacozzo (2009) have noted, local temples also mirrored local creations and were not a simple imitation of their Indian origins (14). Indeed, as historian Laurie Sears (2004), who discusses the shadow play form of *Ramayana*, argues, *Ramayana* has been a site of "contestation and accommodation" in that artists adopted and adapted certain concepts from others to boost their own cultural capital (276). Hence, if an Indian beauty standard traveled to precolonial Java and was adapted to the Javanese context, it was because it made sense to the Javanese people of the time.

However, these sources don't tell us much about the ideal of beauty and the configuration of categories of identities such as skin color and gender in precolonial Java. It is therefore important that I turn to literary texts, without which it would be almost impossible to understand these aspects of precolonial Java. Such a turn to literary texts is also necessary in some ways because written historical documents of the precolonial period are practically nonexistent (Vlekke 1960, 25; Ricklefs 2008/2001, 10–11; Creese 2004, 36). The Old Javanese poems (*kakawin*), folktales, myths, legends, Chinese records, Arab travel writings, and relics are an insightful and practical means for historians to access the undocumented past (H. Sarkar 1970, 4; Creese 2004, 36).

Anthropologist Helen Creese (2004) also endorses this turn to literature for understanding the past. She argues:

> In the absence of the usual tools of the historian's trade, such as narrative histories, censuses, trade records and statistics, and official administrative records, we must look beyond narrow classifications of "historical" and "literary" texts in order to expand our knowledge of the Indonesian past. Rather than recording political events and the historical figures who spearheaded them, this history must instead focus on textual, often literary, representations of social and cultural institutions. (36)

These scholars have paved the way for other scholars to rely on literary texts in constructing a version of the past.

In using literary texts to reach back in time to construct a history of values, I also follow in the methodological footsteps of historian Adrian Vickers (2005) who uses the life and novels of Indonesia's greatest literary author, Pramoedya Ananta Toer, as a thread to narrate a history of modern Indonesia. This method is innovative in that it does not merely use literary analysis to read literary texts but rather uses these texts as a guide to traverse the historical journey of modern Indonesia. Indeed, I intend to do much more than a mere textual analysis of *Ramayana*. Rather, I trace materials related to *Ramayana*, including its historical contexts and textual analyses, to construct a history of gender, skin color, and race during the time *Ramayana* was composed and during the period it circulated in both India and Java. Moreover, I also chart the ways in which *rasa*, affect, and emotion, attached to notions of beauty, are deployed in *Ramayana* to erase, naturalize, and produce historical narratives of difference and social inequality. As such, I construct the past through a critical and creative engagement with literary texts.

Ramayana tells the love story of Rama and his beautiful wife, Sita. Most of the story, however, centers around the war, caused by Sita's beauty, between Rama and the evil dark-skinned King Rawana. The turbulent love story begins when Rama, his brother Laksmana, and Sita are exiled in the forest. When Sita is left alone, Rawana, disguised as a hermit, manages to kidnap her and take her to his palace to try to persuade her to marry him. In his desperate attempts to entice Sita, Rawana makes "illusory heads of king Rama and the hero Laksmana, which looked perfectly exact" (*Ramayana* 403) and brings them to Sita to convince her that her husband is dead. Sita, however, would rather die in fire than marry him. As Rama is winning his war against Rawana's army, his aide, the white monkey

Hanuman, rescues Sita. (Hanuman himself is represented as embodying the color of white, which further exposes the color symbolism embedded in *Ramayana*.) Although the two lovers are reunited, Rama questions Sita's fidelity. To prove her purity Sita chooses to jump into the fire. Because she has indeed been loyal to her husband, Sita is saved from the fire: "They were looking at the fire which flamed up as never before, but suddenly it went out. Ah! Well! She was truly faithful. The pyre had changed into a golden lotus, the fire became the petals and the sweet-smelling smoke of the pollen" (*Ramayana* 659).

The Indian version of *Ramayana* was first told orally and hence there were many versions of the story without an exact date of its original composition. Scholars speculate that it might have been composed anytime between 750 BCE and 200 CE (H. Sarkar 1983, 206; R. Goldman 1984, vol. 1, 23), with most scholars agreeing that *Ramayana* existed prior to the development of Buddhism in India around 500 BCE (Pathak 1968, 128). The most well-known version of the Indian *Ramayana* is attributed to the poet Valmiki, the oldest version of which survived in palm leaf and was dated 1020 CE (Saran and Khanna 2004, 11). This version, however, was composed in Nepal, once again providing evidence for the transnational nature of *Ramayana*.

The Old Javanese version of *Ramayana* was adapted from its Indian origin during King Balitun's reign, around the late ninth to early tenth century (898–930 CE) (Santoso 1980, 17). Because there were many versions of the Indian *Ramayana*, it is not clear from which Indian version of *Ramayana* the Old Javanese *Ramayana* was adapted. Some scholars would argue that the Old Javanese *Ramayana* drew from the *Bhattikavya* version and not from the more popular Indian Valmiki's *Ramayana*, although the author of the Old Javanese version was certainly versed in Valmiki's *Ramayana* (Titib 1998, 31–32; Saran and Khanna 2004, 6). However, not all parts of *Ramayana* were adapted from *Bhattikavya*—only the beginning to the middle of the sixteenth canto were—and it is not clear where the rest of the text came from (H. Sarkar 1983, 210). Tales from *Ramayana* are depicted in sculptures at temples such as Prambanan, Panataran, Siwa, and Brahma around the same period (Chatterji 1967, 81–83; Bandem 1992, 60; Saran and Khana 2004, 20, 32). The tales inscribed on the Shiva temple reliefs were partly influenced by Valmiki's *Ramayana* (Saran and Khanna 2004, 36). I use both *Bhattikavya* and Valmiki's *Ramayana* when discussing the Indian versions of *Ramayana*. I use the English version of *Ramayana*, translated from the Old Javanese by Soewito Santoso,[2] in closely reading the Old Javanese version of *Ramayana*.

My use of the Old Javanese *Ramayana kakawin* is important and arguably even necessary for my purposes for three reasons. First, the Old Javanese *Ramayana* is the oldest surviving major literary work in Indonesia and the "finest" *kakawin* produced in ancient Java (Titib 1998, 29). As a body of work that originated in India and traveled to Java, *Ramayana* functions as a thread with which I stitch together transnational narratives about skin color as it intersects with race and gender from India to precolonial Java. Because the Old Javanese texts are not merely translations but "creative adaptations" of the Indian ones and became their own "original works" (Teeuw 1986, 196)—at least one-third of the Old Javanese *Ramayana* was independent work (Titib 1998, 31)—they may help us understand the ways in which skin color and beauty ideologies traveled from India but then were adapted to a Javanese context. Examining *Ramayana* allows me to chart the transmission and transformation of beauty ideals that are part of transnational circulations of people and ideas.

Second, although the Old Javanese *Ramayana* was a royal court–sponsored text, written for and by the dominant male elite, *Ramayana* was read in public performances and had thus become a popular body of work. It is one of the most popular epic stories in Indonesia and India (Chatterji 1967, 69). In ancient India, *Ramayana* was recited in public both for the purpose of promoting the spiritual welfare of the kings and their people and for political purposes (Saran and Khanna 2004, 10). Some scholars argue that the Indian *Ramayana* was composed to support Aryan civilization (Vyas 1967, 3, 27; A. Sarkar 1987, 11). In the Indian *Ramayana*, Rama is represented as taking part in the dissemination of Aryan culture in south India (A. Sarkar 1987, 8). In precolonial Indonesia, *Ramayana* was used to revive the religious teachings of Hinduism because around the seventh century Buddhism had become a strong influence in Sumatra and West and Central Java (Sunoto 1992, 50). So dominant was the influence of these Indian-origin Old Javanese texts that even to the present day this influence still persists, and in most places in Java heroes from popular Old Javanese texts continue to be more popular than Islamic ones (Creese 2004, 23–24; Zoetmulder 1974, 23). It is its popularity and political significance that render *Ramayana* an influential text.

Third, as a utopian text that projected an ideal world, *Ramayana* provided a way for people to imagine the world as it "should" be (J. Taylor 2003, 44; Creese 2004, 5, 23, 42). This, as well as the fact that beauty discourse is so prominent in the *kakawins* genre (Creese 2004, 28), allows us to consider the Old Javanese texts valid sources for understanding the female beauty ideal in that period. A word of caution is necessary: the Old Javanese text that I discuss here can only help us understand the *discourse* of women's beauty and not necessarily the preferences of "real" people. With such a disclaimer, I do not argue that the "real" world and the world of "representation" are two distinct and separate worlds. As cultural studies scholar Raymond Williams has pointed out, "art reflects its society. . . . But also, art creates, by new perceptions and responses, elements which the society, as such, is not able to realize. If we compare art with its society, we find a series of real relationships showing its deep and central connections with the rest of the general life" (2009, 42). What Williams hinted at here, which I also embrace, is that art can be examined to reveal different aspects of reality. Art is but one expression of "reality." Hence examining a work of art can help us understand a certain aspect of society that we may overlook if we were only to look at real lives.

Finally, *Ramayana* is a beautifully written poem filled with rich emotions. Hence, this chapter, as it relies on emotions as a lens through which it senses and narrates the history of the past finds *Ramayana* to be a perfect site for its analysis.

RASA AS A LENS TO SENSE AND CENSOR HISTORY: FEELING AND PEELING THE DIFFERENT LAYERS OF REALITY

Rasa is not the same as affect nor can it be reduced to affect or emotion. *Rasa* was constructed based on a "psychological analysis of the human mind in ancient times" (Nandi 1973, 233). As literary scholar R. Patankar carefully notes, "when we study a conceptual structure like the *rasa* theory across many centuries, we find that it contains parts which are completely unintelligible to us, and others which possess only historical interest" (1986, 110). *Rasa* is thus an appropriate tool for the purpose of examining the text produced during this precolonial time. However, I develop the concept of *rasa* by putting *rasa*, affect, and emotion into productive conversation. Thus, although I draw from theories of *rasa* produced by scholars of ancient India and Java, I also make use of theories of affect and emotion circulated in the United States.

In the Indian context, the concept of *rasa* is confined within the realm of the artistic and aesthetic worlds of dance and dramatic performance and is often framed as being in tension with and disconnected from the real world—indeed, as a feeling that cannot be experienced in ordinary life (Nandi 1986, 43; 1973, 364; Ambardekar 1979, 30). As Sanskrit scholar René Daumal explains, *rasa* "is not related to the ordinary 'world'; it is a recreation of that 'world' on another plane. . . . It is not 'of this world'" (1970/1982, 12). *Rasa*, then, is "an *imitation* of feelings and moods realized through inference with the help of unfailing marks in the actor" (Nandi 1986, 46; emphasis mine). The concept of imitation in *rasa* once again highlights the performativity of *rasa*: the performer has to success-fully imitate or perform a particular feeling in order for the audience to relish the essence of that emotion, or that *rasa*. *Rasa*, in this sense, is performance-bound: *rasa* can only be felt for as long as the performance takes place and does not continue beyond that performance (Kulkarni 1986, 31). *Rasa* is then the feeling that the audience experiences when savoring the emotional content of a work of art; it is also the emotion that dominates a work of art (Higgins 2007, 44, 50; Walton 2007, 32).

Not all spectators, however, can automatically experience *rasa* when watching a performance. There are various factors that must work together in order for the audience to experience *rasa*. The first one is the determinant (*vibhavas*), defined as "the causes of emotion, such as elements in a drama that might bring forth old memories and rouse the emotions"; the second is consequent (*anubhava*), understood as "the physical effects (for example, blushing) arising due to the determinants"; the third is "complementary psychological states (*vyabhicaribhava*)," the "secondary, transient emotions, such as weeping with joy" (Walton 2007, 32). In addition to these three factors, the audience must be able to "transcend his or her ego, [and] merg[e] completely with the work of art" to experience *rasa* (2007, 32). It is this suspension of ego that allows the "sensitive" audience to transform *bhava* (emotion felt in "ordinary" life) into *rasa*. This transformation is made possible when a sensitive audience attends to their "affective trajectory." Higgins explains, "the elements of resuscitated memory enable one who experiences an artwork or other affect-producing stimuli to recognize the convergence of one's own experience and the emotion one encounters in another" (Higgins 2007, 47–49; quote on 48). For example, as she suggested, an adult could relate to a child's emotion by remembering his or her own childhood experiences. We rely on these "deposited memory elements" found within our affective trajectory to make sense of feelings experienced at a particular moment. Hence, *rasa* is accessed through "the stimulation . . . of previously deposited memory elements . . . , which are transmitted by [the poet's suggestive] words" (Higgins 2007, 47). *Rasa* is something that is "suggested" and not directly stated (Walton 2007, 32–33). Additionally, to experience *rasa*, the audience must be a "cultured" audience (Higgins 2007, 46). This means that just as only *gourmands* can really savor the exquisite taste of gourmet food (Kulkarni 1986, 8), only sensitive and cultured audiences can relish the *rasa* of a work of art. This aspect of *rasa* suggests that emotions are socially constructed: they must be learned and cultivated (Reddy 2001, 59).

The Indian version of *rasa* thus allows us to understand how we produce affective responses to a stimulus that we know is not real. That is, when we watch a performance such as *Ramayana* we know that

> the actor who is personifying Rama is not Rama. Thus what appears is false. But one does not see it in this way. Similarly, one does not doubt whether the actor is or is not Rama. Nor one [sic] has the knowledge of the actor's similarity with Rama. So, none of the logical modes of knowledge holds good [sic] of this experience and yet there is a real experience (*sphurannanubhavah*). So,

in what way is this throbbing experience be [*sic*] understood? . . . The point to be noted here is that . . . the experience of the creation of imagination is real in its own right, even though, it may not fall under any recognized logical category. (Nandi 1973, 363)

Rasa is therefore a useful tool because as a mode of feeling it helps us understand how emotions about "unreal" or "performative" characters can be felt and with what consequences. As a theoretical concept, *rasa* also helps us comprehend why different individuals might respond differently to the same performative events, characters, images, or representations: the audience's affective response to literary texts or performances depends on their affective trajectory and previously deposited memory elements. Thus no one can guarantee whether or not the audience will savor *rasa*. This further emphasizes the audience's or the reader's agency.

In the Javanese context, *rasa* encompasses the artistic as well as the spiritual worlds. Anthropologist Clifford Geertz has pointed out, "*rasa* is the 'connecting link' between the three major components of religious life: mystical practice, art, and etiquette" (quoted in Walton 2007, 33). Ethnomusicologist Marc Benamou, in the context of Java, defines *rasa* as "an extrasensory faculty of perception, through which the properly trained heart can 'feel' essences directly" (2010, 50). Moreover, *rasa* signifies a sense of awareness "*through* feeling" and not necessarily awareness "*of* feeling" (Stange 1984, 119). Ethnomusicologist Susan Walton clarifies that "as 'feeling,' [*rasa*] refers to the physical senses of taste and touch and also to emotional feelings. . . . *Rasa* can mean the essential, often hidden, significance of something obscure. . . . For the Javanese, to fathom something obscure, one has to engage all one's senses, feelings, and intuitions, as if one were tasting the essence of the thing. To use merely one's intellectual capacities is not enough" (2007, 31). Hence, the concept of *rasa* helps us understand how knowledge can be produced *through* feeling. For example, as I will discuss later in this chapter, we can learn about skin color hierarchies in precolonial Java as articulated in a discourse concerning beauty *through* the feeling of fear evoked by the dark-skinned characters in *Ramayana* such as King Rawana.

In both Indian and Javanese contexts, *rasa* registers as "an experience at once physical, emotional, and cognitive" (Schwartz 2004, 50). Physical reactions provide us with clues as to which emotions we are feeling. These physical reactions, *rasa* theorist G. K. Bhat points out, "bring the emotion to the level of perception or consciousness of an observer; so that what was determined by the presence of the stimulating cause is now perceptibly clear, as it were, due to the physical consequences plainly and vividly manifested" (1984, 12). In a sense, *rasa* functions like affect in that *rasa* has a physical dimension and is understood as "physical activities" (Ambardekar 1979, 131). An example that feminist studies scholar

Elspeth Probyn (2005), in the Australian context, uses in her discussion of affect as having physical properties is blushing, which is a physical manifestation of shame, a physical clue that informs us that we are feeling shame. Similarly, *rasa*, like affect, relies on the importance of the body. In the Old Javanese *Ramayana*, the body is thought of as "the instrument we play on. It is full of happy and sad tunes, and so it was and [always] will be" (*Ramayana* 709). Thus, the body is an important site, an "instrument," if you will, through which we access our *rasa*.

However, in carefully understanding the meaning of the body in accessing our feelings, there is a difference between *rasa* and affect. That is, unlike affect, which exists prior to moments of cognition, as philosophers Brian Massumi (2002) and Gilles Deleuze and Félix Guattari (1987) have all pointed out, *rasa* is experienced cognitively. The cognitive aspect of *rasa* should not simply be understood in terms of being registered purely in the mind, however. Rather, *rasa* is also registered by the body. Anthropologist Kalpana Ram (2000) offers the concept of "synaesthesia of the senses" to name the phenomenon of how the body responds in certain patterns when hearing or seeing specific artistic performances because these stimuli evoke the body's physical memory. This concept can be likened to "muscle memory": the ways in which the body remembers how to move after much dance practice. Hence, here the body registers the event even when the mind may not consciously recognize it. Taking this concept of "synaesthesia of the senses" to issues of race, gender, and the construction of skin color, I point to the ways in which a "synaesthesia of the senses" operates when we construct race, color, and gender in our lives. When our body encounters other bodies, we may be more likely to have bodily responses that reflect certain affective patterns because of how our memory is being evoked and shaped by previous encounters, which need not be "real" encounters. Some "technologies of memories," which according to postcolonial scholar Pamela Pattynama include "films, objects, representations and also bodies" (2007, 70), help shape how our bodies respond when seeing beautiful people, for example.

Sensing and Making Sense of History

In both versions of *Ramayana*, the Indian and the Old Javanese, beautiful women are described in similar ways. What is interesting about the way beautiful women are described in these precolonial texts is the use of specific metaphors in relation to brightness or light, such as the moon. In the Old Javanese *Ramayana*, the protagonist's wife, Sita, is described as having a "white shining" face that is likened to the full moon (Titib 1998, 97; *Ramayana* 225). For example, in one of the episodes when the monkey troop finds Sita, she is described as a "young maiden, truly beautiful and well behaved. She shone like the moon"

(*Ramayana* 188). Moreover, in endearingly remembering his wife who is kidnapped by Rawana, Rama agonizes:

> My memory of your sweet look is kindled by the sight of a deer, the elephant reminds me of your elegance, the moon of your brilliant face. Ah! I am possessed by your beauty. (*Ramayana* 178)

In the Old Javanese *Ramayana*, the moon is often evoked to represent women's complexional beauty. As the evil King Dasamukha encounters Sita, he asks, "Who are you, o beautiful one, who enters the forest to pick flowers. How unparalleled is your beauty, most perfect. Even the beauty of the moon is no match for yours, because it waned at daytime and becomes ugly without radiance" (*Ramayana* 122). It is clear that it is the moon's radiant, bright, and shining properties that are likened to women's beauty, but the moon pales in comparison to Sita's beauty because the moon wanes and therefore loses its radiance. Thus when Hanuman finds Sita after she has been taken hostage by Rawana, her face does not shine anymore: "[Dust] had covered her shiny white face, like the full moon dimmed by haze" (*Ramayana* 225). Moreover, when the evil king's sister raksasi[3] Surpanaka seduces Rama's brother, Laksmana, she "took another form, she became perfect in beauty, [her face was] like the full moon" (*Ramayana* 95).

In the Indian *Ramayana*, the moon is the author's favorite metaphor, one to which he returns often in describing the beautiful qualities of certain characters, days, situations, or things. The moon[4] is also used to compare things that have white, bright, and shining colors such as necklaces, chariots, and umbrellas as well as to describe one's psychological state positively. The moon is certainly the most common metaphor used to describe women's beauty. However, the moon, especially in its waxing state, does not represent any and all kinds of beauty. As Sanskrit scholar Madhusudan Pathak argues, the full moon is a common metaphor used in old literary works to describe the "excellence of the beauty of the complexion," the "complexional beauty," or the "beauty and brilliance of a woman" (1968, 25–26, 41, quotes from 32, 34–35, 100). The focus on metaphor is related to the fact that metaphor is used very frequently in *Ramayana*. In the Indian *Ramayana*, it is used every eighth or tenth line (Pathak 1968, 13). The moon is the most frequent metaphor used in *Ramayana*, along with the sun and fire.

Such evocation of beauty functions to arouse people's desires. That is, the moon stands for beauty because, as scholar of mythology Jules Cashford points out, "in earlier times with nothing but stars, fires and candles to light up the night, the Moon must have been overwhelming" (2003, 272). It may be this overwhelming feeling of seeing the moon that was likened to the overwhelming feeling of seeing the face of a beautiful woman. Similarly, in the Indian context, as Pathak points out, "the sky is usually clear and bright. The sun and the moon shine brightly on most of the days and nights. So these two brilliant luminaries perpetually present before the eyes of a creator of literature, are quite likely to inspire in him a *feeling* of wonder at the realization of the *indescribable beauty* which they possess" (1968, 29; emphasis mine). In the Old Javanese context, Bhat suggests, "pleasure-garden, moon, spring season and such other factors . . . excite and strengthen the particular emotion roused by the stimulating cause" (1984, 11–12). The moon is therefore used in these poems because it can incite certain emotions and have particular consequences: desire toward beautiful characters of a particular skin color and gender.

This method of evoking an object to articulate certain emotions, according to British poet T. S. Eliot, is related to the fact that "emotion cannot be expressed directly, but has to be conveyed through 'objective correlatives'" (quoted in Bhat 1984, 60). Eliot points out:

> The only way of expressing emotion in the form of art is by finding an objective correlative, in other words, a set of objects which shall be the formula of that *particular* emotion, so that when the external facts, which must turn in sensory experience, are given, the emotion is immediately evoked. (1932/1958, 145)

Following this logic, I argue that the full moon in these texts is deployed to suggest a particular *rasa* such as love toward beautiful women. Particularly because in these texts beautiful women are sites where love, romance, and desire take place, the moon that in the north Indian myth "constitutes the legendary source of all interpersonal attraction, love, romance and desire" makes a reasonable comparison with beauty (Abbi 2002, 512). Indeed, in these texts, women's beauty is represented to arouse "pangs of love" (*Ramayana* 720) or as "the stirrer of the heart stirred up, as it were, my whole heart" (Meyer 2003, 280–281).

Clearly, the moon, signifying women's beauty, does the work of stimulating a particular *rasa*, that of love, toward the subjects described as beautiful. This is because emotion does the work of "moving" people. Bhat points out,

> A poet writes in order to express or communicate an intensely moving emotional experience; he [*sic*] is in the role of a *bhavayita* or one who wants to bring about something. He wants that his communication should reach the reader and make him respond; this is *bhavir* or something intended to happen. His writing, the poetic or dramatic composition, is then the *bhavaka* or an instrument of the intended communication and of affective result. The writer's creative effort, which includes the significant form he

imposes on the emotional experience, the literary graces of presentation, all the devices to attract the reader favourably towards the writing, may be regarded as an operation favourable to the intended happening (*bhavana-anukula-vyapara*). (1984, 37)

Hence, the production of *rasa* matters because it can function as an instrument that drives readers toward an intended happening. In other words, *rasa* can move people, their feelings and actions. Here, I am referring to this feeling as *rasa* because this feeling of love or desire toward the character is not "real" as such and ceases to exist once the reader finishes reading the text. This feeling of love is not a permanent or real emotion. To argue that this feeling is not a real emotion is not to argue that that feeling does not register in the reality of the viewer's life. Rather, this feeling is felt at a different layer of reality. This feeling is then deposited as part of that person's affective trajectory and body memory. In future encounters, these deposited memory elements could, when evoked, produce certain affective responses.

These affective evocations toward beautiful women produce what Probyn calls "affective scripts" (2005, 23). Psychologist Silvan Tomkins frames "script theory" to chart the ways in which a person would interpret and respond to an event according to a specific "scene" and the relationship between scenes (148). Probyn, drawing from Tomkins' work, defines "affective scripts" as the ways in which "the human organism incorporates in an intimate way early affective scenes. Disparate bits of information become script or theory, which interact with the work of parts of the brain and the nervous system" (23). She further clarifies, "if individual women have experienced early in their lives primal scenes of shame and humiliation, seeing other women shamed will tend to reactivate the feeling" (84). What she underlines here is that it is the ways in which our feelings are reactivated when encountering familiar scenes that constitute affective scripts. However, unlike Probyn and Tomkins who appropriately situate affective scripts within one's real life for the cases they examine, I take affective scripts beyond real life application and apply them to these different layers of reality: both the real and the imaginary world. This means that I find affective scripts useful for discussing feelings that are reactivated when encountering "scenes" in literature or films as well as in real life. Stories such as *Ramayana* provide people with affective scripts of how we should feel toward certain performative subjects and events.

Indeed, throughout this epic poem, many metaphors are used to highlight the ways in which white is affectively represented as desirable for its attachment to beauty, purity, and cleanliness. The pollen of pandanus in the Old Javanese *Ramayana* is used as "face powder, so that [the women] look perfectly white" (*Ramayana* 697). When the King Dasanana comes to kidnap Sita, he disguises himself as a hermit and is described as having "teeth [that] were very clean and white like crystals" (*Ramayana* 121). When the ascetic whose skin is turned black asks Rama to turn her skin back into her natural color, she says, "touch my face with your hand. Let it be you who puts a complete end to the curse befalling me. Deliver me from my impurity" (*Ramayana* 150). Even flowers are described as being "so pure and white, as if they were smiling" (*Ramayana* 399). In all of these examples, purity and whiteness are attached to signifiers of positive *rasa* and physical expressions such as smiles. Moreover, radiance and beauty are also attached to beautiful feelings: to lift Rama's sadness, "the Moon (god) came up gloriously to [*sic*] eastern mountain with radiance and beauty, as if he wanted to comfort [Rama] when he saw him mourning" (*Ramayana* 308).

What is interesting, however, is affective scripts that are imbued with and expressed through discourses of gender and skin color. Throughout both versions of *Ramayana*, evil characters are described as having dark skin color and are represented through objective correlatives that symbolize darkness and suggest some negative *rasas*. First, black and dark skin color is used to suggest the *rasa* of suffering. In the Old Javanese *Ramayana*, a lady ascetic whose skin is as "black as the colour of collyrium" (*Ramayana* 97–98, 148) narrates how her skin changes its color to black as a form of punishment when she eats the flesh of the God Wisnu. She sees her transformation to black skin as "the origin of her suffering" (*Ramayana* 150). This deployment of darkness to mark one's suffering can also be seen in another scene in which the protagonist's wife, Sita, is sad when she is separated from her husband. In this scene she is represented "like the moon at the dark fortnight because of her sufferings" (*Ramayana* 300). Darkness and dark skin, therefore, are conflated in these scenes through the *rasa* of suffering.

Worthy to note in this epic poem is the ways in which darkness is attached to nighttime and how both darkness and nighttime are attached to negative *rasas*. Sadness, for example, is linked to darkness: "Sad is the heart of the pessimist who sees only darkness all around, darkness that in no way will lift" (*Ramayana* 175). Moreover, when Rama articulates his sadness at being away from Sita, he laments,

> At daytime I do not long a great deal, I see many things in the woods that heal, at nighttime I am lost in affliction, aimlessly my mind wanders without direction. . . . I wish that the night would be brief, and it always daytime be. Ah, I am weak and in grief, at night the memory of you is haunting me. (*Ramayana* 179)

Nighttime as representing darkness is also associated with evil and wandering demons. Says the king of the monkeys Sugriwa to his troops: "there are many wild demons roaming there at night-time" (*Ramayana* 185). These examples suggest how darkness and nighttime are used to signify negative *rasas* such as fear or sadness.

Moreover, people with dark/black skin are mentioned in the texts to affectively signify fear. In the Old Javanese *Ramayana*, the affective vocabularies that surround the concept of darkness and therefore provide affective signifiers for darkness, are words such as "dangerous," "terrifying," and "doom." Indeed, at the end the dark-complexioned king and his troops are doomed to death. A few more examples of how dark-skinned people, the "evil" king and his people, are represented in the Old Javanese *Ramayana* will suffice to illustrate this point:

On King Dasasya: "his black complexion made him look like the flashing clouds of doom." (*Ramayana* 329)

On King Dasamuka's troops: "Their bodies were black-skinned, muscular and strong, like a very dangerous mountain. Their mustaches were thick and black like rain clouds, their canine teeth sharp like lightning. Their eyes started from their sockets, round and glowing like the sun shining with a thousand rays, hot like flaming fire. Their eyebrows were entangled, like smoke whirling up." (*Ramayana* 258)

King Rawana's attendants are described as "looking terrifying and black like rain clouds, their swords resembling flashes of lightning." (*Ramayana* 538)

King Rawana is depicted thus: "The king [Rawana] looked at [his brother] with loving eyes, but his glance was frightful. He was equal to a venomous snake, his deeds gave fright to everyone [seeing him]." (*Ramayana* 334)

These examples show a consistent pattern of the ways in which dark-skinned people are represented by metaphors of nature deemed dangerous, such as the "rain clouds." These objects are the "objective correlatives . . . through which emotional experience is to be expressed" (Bhat 1984, 19–20). Here, it is not simply the property of the dark cloud that is being compared to the king's dark skin. Rather, it is the *feeling* of being terrified when the dark rain cloud hangs low during a thunderstorm, that is being likened to the *feeling* of encountering these dark-skinned people. Hence, what happens here is the conflation of the darkness of the cloud with darkness of one's skin, which is registered through the production of feeling or *rasa*. Thus, it is important that the cloud is specified as the dark rain cloud and not the wispy white cloud, because the dark cloud as is the case in Western literary tradition, has been used to reinforce a "dark" mood (Wilson 1983, 21). The fear of blackness may even be rooted "in the child's horror of the night—a time of isolation, disturbing dreams, and nightmares, when invisibility of the familiar encourages fantasy to run wild" (Gergen 1967, quoted in Tuan 1974/1990, 25). Race and Japanese studies scholar Hiroshi Wagatsuma also made an interesting observation when he pointed out that dark-skinned Africans were visually represented in Japan *after* Buddhist mythology's devils and demons (1967, 413). In other words, the process of demonizing dark-skinned people relied on the pre-existing darkness-as-evil concept. It is not simply that dark-skinned people were attached to negative affects and therefore demonized. Rather, if dark-skinned people were represented as evil characters, it might be because it made sense for people fearful of the darkness existing in nature and their lives to begin with.

In addition to being affectively represented as dangerous and fearsome, darkness is also depicted as an abject entity, needing to be eliminated. In the Indian *Ramayana*, "the cool-rayed moon is rising, dispelling the darkness of the world and gladdening with his radiance the hearts of all its creatures" (R. Goldman 1984, 189). Similarly, in the Old Javanese *Ramayana*, when "the moon came up . . . darkness fled away, like the demons fleeing away at the approach of god Hari" (*Ramayana* 210). Darkness is represented as inferior to light: when the light comes, it chases the darkness away.

This perception of darkness as undesirable represents the color symbolism of that early pre-European colonial period.[5] Color has indeed been used to symbolize social differentiation in ancient societies (Thapar 2002, 29–30). In ancient India, white was considered a lucky color to be presented to the gods, while red, which signified "evil magic" or death, along with black were ones to be offered to the evil spirits (*bhuta*) (Meyer 2003, 266 fn. 2). Moreover, a Brahman woman in ancient India who slept with a man of a different caste would have to be dragged along the street naked with an appropriate color of a donkey (black donkey for a Çudra, lower-caste man, yellow for a Vaiçya man, white for an upper-caste Kshattriya man) to be cleansed of her sin (Meyer 2003, 255 fn. 1). Moreover, colors are embedded within Indian emotive archetypes. They are used to express the "emotive states in costuming and makeup as visual cues: white is related to humor, whereas black symbolizes fear and panic" (Schwartz 2004, 15–16).

All of these suggest that using *rasa* as a lens to read *Ramayana* is productive in gauging the colorism at work in precolonial India and Java. Employing *rasa* allows me to show how dark-skinned people are represented to affectively signify negative feelings. This highlights that the purpose of this chapter is not simply to demonstrate the representation of dark-skinned people as "evil" characters and light-skinned women as beautiful. Rather, the analysis is intended to show how the production of *rasas* is attached to, made possible by, and revealing of a colorism that existed in precolonial Indian and Javanese societies.

To make *rasa*, affect, and emotions visible in narratives is therefore to better understand how *rasa* works in shaping our history. Storytelling and history telling are part of affective production. Indeed, when *Ramayana* was recited, people felt the circuit of vibrations (Saran and Khanna 2004, 9). Hence, how we tell our history matters. It matters because our stories inevitably contribute to the production of affective scripts that we tell about people, places, and events. Although I have pointed out the danger in how certain emotions can be deployed to naturalize gender and color hierarchies, this chapter is *not* a call for constructing a history that is free from *rasa* or emotions. Rather, the call here is to make visible how *rasa*, or the underlying emotions that help us shape our sense of reality, works as an apparatus of ideology even as we tell our own version of history. After all, all stories, including history, are colored by certain *rasa*.

BY WAY OF CONCLUSION: CENSORED HISTORY, ERASING AND RACE-ING HISTORY

All texts, as philosopher Judith Butler argues, experience some forms of censorship. One form of censorship occurs at the level of the author when the author decides what to write based on the author's sense of what can be written (1997b, 133). The author's *sense* of the event, and I would further argue how she *feels* about the event, shapes which stories are written and how these stories are written. Adoration for our heroes, for example, is written in and through history. In fact, heroes and heroines are not inherently important figures prior to the process of narrativization and historicization (Kasetsiri 2003, 13). They *become* heroes and heroines in the moment of our telling their stories. In this sense, history becomes a narrative that could normalize and naturalize the feelings we have for these historical events and characters.

Rasa, I thus argue, matters in shaping historical narratives insofar as certain degrees of romanticization of the precolonial period erase traces of color hierarchies existing in this period. This means that positive feelings about the precolonial period may move us to paint a rosy picture and disregard colorism operating within the beauty discourse. Hence, my point here is that feelings matter in how historians capture, that is to say "censor," history.

In the Indonesian context, discussions of racism often frame the colonial period as the historical moment during which racism emerged (Gouda 1995; Stoler 2002; J. Taylor 2003). What has been missing from these discussions is the ways in which colorism shaped how racism was carried out in colonial Indonesia and that this had already taken hold in the minds of people in the archipelago prior to European colonialism. In other words, when the European colonizers arrived in Indonesia, they arrived in a place where light skin color was already discursively valued and considered as the beauty ideal. The colonizer, as I will discuss in chapter two, certainly shifted the meaning of light skin color and conflated it with "race." Nonetheless, the seed of preference for light skin color already existed during precolonial Java as we have seen in the Old Javanese adaptation of the Indian epic poem *Ramayana*.

I have developed the concept of *rasa* and deployed it as a theoretical-emotional lens to sense and censor history. Employing *rasa* as a lens to sense the reality of the past allows me to argue that preference for women with light skin color already existed prior to European colonization, and that the preference for light-skinned women in women's beauty discourse was maintained and circulated across various geographical locations. My argument challenges dominant historical narratives of precolonial India and precolonial Java as ideal and idyllic times and places, and also challenges the conception that colorism is rooted in European colonialism.

I also argue that conflation between lightness and light skin as desirable and darkness and dark skin as undesirable is registered through *rasa*. *Rasa* (and its theoretical frame of reference, "affects") does the work of categorizing certain women as more beautiful than others in precolonial Java. Indeed, the mechanism deployed in these texts to affectively produce beautiful subjects as desirable subjects is the conflation between the positive *rasa* produced by evoking metaphors of lightness, brightness, and radiance such as the moon whose meanings are desirable, beautiful, and pure, and the positive *rasa* attached to these beautiful women. Simultaneously, the meanings such as evil, undesirable, and ugly, attached to metaphors of darkness is transferred, stands for, and provides meanings for *rasa* suggested by the darkness of skin color. In both versions of *Ramayana*, the full moon (or other correlative objects) is used affectively and effectively to evoke positive *rasa* toward these beautiful women. This is problematic when standards of beauty are articulated through discourses of gender and skin color (and as we'll see, race) and is used to naturalize and hide social hierarchies embedded in such beauty norms.

The preference for light skin color during this period, however, should not be read as preference for Caucasian white skin color. During precolonial time, the specificity that links lightness (of skin color) and whiteness (of race) had not yet been established. This may have been because race as we refer to it today did not exist then. As literary scholar Robert Young argues:

> We can say that explicit theorizations of race began in the late eighteenth century, were increasingly scientized in the nineteenth, and came to an official end as an ideology after 1945 with the UNESCO statements about

race (which is not to say that they did not continue in theory or in practice). Racial theory cannot be separated from its own historical moment: it was developed at a particular era of British and European colonial expansion in the nineteenth century which ended in the Western occupation of nine-tenths of the surface territory of the globe. (1995, 91)

Thus, we must take into account that skin color during the late ninth and early tenth centuries had not yet intersected with race as we know it today. This link, or the conflation between race and skin color, only came later. It was indeed during the Dutch colonial period that the meanings of light skin color as the beauty ideal began to be transformed and conflated with race.

2 | Rooting and Routing Whiteness in Colonial Indonesia

From Dutch to Japanese Whiteness

Beauty may come in different shapes, but apparently not in different shades. At least this is what images of beauty that circulated in early- to mid-twentieth-century Indonesia would seem to suggest. If during the precolonial era the brightness of the moon functioned as an objective correlative for beauty, in early- to mid-twentieth-century Indonesia what appeared on the pages of women's magazines were the beautiful faces of different races of women models—Caucasian, Japanese, Indonesian—but all white.

Tracing the shifts in beauty ideals during the colonial period, I will focus solely on the emergence of two categories of whiteness: "European whiteness" and "Japanese whiteness." The formation of "Indonesian whiteness" as part of the postcolonial nation's struggle in articulating its gendered national identity against these "white" colonial powers will be discussed in the next chapter. Here I show how circulations of people and ideas from the Netherlands and Japan engendered particular beauty ideals in colonial Indonesia and that what counted as light skin throughout these periods differed significantly over time.

Examining the historical emergence of these two categories of whiteness, I make visible not only the complex construction of multiple categories of whiteness that emerged as a result of transnational circulations of people and ideas in Indonesia but also the shift that happened during these two colonial periods: from attempts to *conflate* skin color with race to attempts to *dissociate* these two categories of identity, and the intricate and subtle ways the ideology of emotion helped shape these processes of identity formation. In the Dutch colonial period that peaked during 1900–1942, it was light-skinned Caucasian women who were considered the epitome of beauty. This process of representing Caucasian women as the face of beauty highlights the ways in which racial projects of colonialism were successful in their attempt to conflate skin color with race. I use racial projects here as race scholars Michael Omi and Howard Winant define them: *"simultaneously an interpretation, representation, or explanation of racial dynamics, and an effort to reorganize and redistribute resources along particular racial lines"* (1994, 56; emphasis original). This conflation between skin color and race was meant to create a distinct white skin color/racial category in which only Caucasians would be positioned in the white skin color/racial category. An example from the late-eighteenth-century Chinese context might help explain this better: although up to that period both Chinese and Europeans had been considered "whites," Europeans argued that their "superiority" over the Chinese must mean they had different skin colors. Europeans then claimed to be the sole possessor of white skin and designated yellow as the color of Chinese skin (Demel 2001, 36). In colonial Indonesia, the process of marking Europeans as the only racial group that could occupy the racial/skin color "white" category was only successful in beauty discourse, however. Beyond beauty discourse, the boundary of who could be considered racially white *and* white-skinned was unclear; racial projects that were implemented in colonial Indonesia actually produced a white racial category that only partly relied on skin color as its signifier. It is crucial that the particularity of the Indonesian experience of racial formation under colonialism be noted. During this period, some dark-skinned Javanese could request and be granted "European equivalence"; the Japanese were even regarded as "honorary Europeans." Both examples demonstrated how the boundary of the white skin color/racial category was anything but definitive.

This messy racial and skin color configuration was further complicated when Japanese colonization (1942–1945) challenged the Caucasian white beauty ideal. Not only did the Japanese challenge the Caucasian white beauty ideal by replacing it with an Asian one, but they also challenged the belief that Caucasians were the sole possessors of white skin by claiming that Asians could appropriate and even own white skin. It is important to remember that although in the United States the word yellow has been used to signify "Asian" race, Asians have used other words to describe their skin color. The Japanese, for example, use the word "shiroi," which means white and is the same word used for white paper and snow, and white skin color in general, to describe their own skin color (Wagatsuma 1967, 411). This notion that Asians could also possess white skin color underscores the ways in which skin color was dissociated from race: people could have white skin color but they did not necessary belong to the white racial group. This attempt to dissociate race from skin color, however, failed in practice because the Japanese own understanding of skin color at the time was already one that was infused with Western white ideals—the dissociation of race from skin color, as I will discuss in chapter five, was more successful in post-Independence Indonesia.

To provide a historical overview of the place of skin color in constructing women's beauty discourse during the colonial and postcolonial periods, I draw extensively from memoirs, newspapers, women's magazines, and especially advertisements relating to women's beauty and skin-whitening products in early- to mid-twentieth-century Indonesia. Examining beauty advertisements and beauty columns published in women's magazines and other periodicals is necessary to provide an understanding of the dominant discourse of beauty as it was articulated and visualized in popular media during that time. Analyzing *images* of beauty is even more important for this period when most of the population were illiterate. I am aware, however, that the "reality" was more convoluted than the representations in these magazines. Nonetheless, this is precisely why looking at the beauty discourse as it was represented in magazines allows me to understand the beauty *ideal* at the time. As in the present moment, for example, the supermodels represented in magazines do not necessarily depict the reality of most women in the world. These representations are revealing of the dominant race, gender, and skin color ideology of our contemporary time.

Among the periodicals that I examine are *Bintang Hindia* (1928), *De Huisvrouw in Deli* (1933, 1935), *Keng Po* (1933, 1938), *Pewarta Arab* (1933), *De Huisvrouw in Indie* (1933, 1936–1937, 1940–1941), *Vereniging van Huisvrouwen Cheribon* (1936), *Fu Len* (1938), *De Huisvrouw* (1938–1939), *De Huisvrouw in Nord Sumatra* (1939–1940), *Almanak Asia Raya* (1943), *Soeara Asia* (1943–1944), and *Djawa Baroe* (1943–1945). These periodicals were published for local consumption, mostly in cities on the islands of Sumatra and Java.

ROOTING WHITENESS: CAUCASIAN WHITE AS THE BEAUTY IDEAL DURING THE APOGEE OF DUTCH COLONIALISM (1900–1942)

Here I specifically chose to examine the final decades of Dutch colonial rule when colonialism fully matured. Although Dutch colonial settlers had begun to live and interracially reproduce with Javanese and other women prior to the twentieth century, because my main concern is to look at beauty discourses as represented in women's magazines and newspapers, I limit my historical excavation to the peak of colonialism for a couple of reasons. First, after the mid-nineteenth century and after the opening of the Suez Canal, more European women were allowed to migrate to the archipelago, hence allowing for more dynamic interracial relations. Second, after the implementation of the ethical policy in 1901 that allowed some privileged natives access, albeit limited, to education, these natives then became the founders and readers of these magazines. I will expand on these ideas below, but first I will provide a historical context to better understand the archipelago and its ever-changing communities.

Before Europeans arrived in the Indonesian archipelago in the early sixteenth century (Portuguese first, the Dutch a century later), race or ethnicity (not necessarily skin color) had had little significance. It does not mean that in colonial Indonesia or the "Dutch East Indies" (Indies) there had existed only racial homogeneity and no racial differences. On the contrary, in addition to some Europeans, Abyssinians, Armenians, Arabs, Ambonese, Bengali, Burmese, Bugis, Ceylonese, Chinese, Goans, Gujerati, Javanese, Macassarese, Malabarese, Malays, Persians, Portuguese, Sinhalese, Tamils, Timorese, and Vietnamese had all resided on the islands of the vast archipelago (Blussé 1986, 19; J. Taylor 1992, 249; Colombijn 2000, 44). Yet, race and ethnicity simply indicated the places where people came from, and were made visible by the types of merchandise they sold, the kinds of dress they wore, the languages they spoke, or the cultural traditions they practiced (Colombijn 2000, 45–46).

To explain this lack of ethnic- or race-based identity in the Indies prior to the heyday of Dutch colonialism, scholars have identified several factors. One explanation is that a "cultural blending" took place among Indonesian slaves that weakened ethnic loyalty (Raben 1996, 171). Another explanation looks back to a sixteenth-century period when in Sumatra and Malaca it was the attachment to the king/sultan rather than ethnicity that bound people's loyalty (Colombijn 2000, 44). Finally, another factor may have been the importance of religion rather than ethnicity that at least until the early nineteenth century functioned as a marker of social distinction (Blussé 1986, 5; Mandal 1994, 74; Raben 1996, 263; Fasseur 1997, 32).

Most Indonesians (about 90 percent) identify as Muslim, making it—as U.S. media are quick to point out—the largest Muslim country in the world. It is important, however, that we understand the particularities of Islam in Indonesia. I will explain here a couple of conditions that contribute to such particularities. First, the dominant religions and belief systems in Indonesia prior to the coming of Islam and Christianity were Hinduism, Buddhism, and various local animistic religions (Ropi 2000, 1–2). Hinduism might have existed in Java since the first century CE (Djamaris 1984, 16), although it was around the seventh century when we see evidence of not only Hinduism but also Buddhism in the archipelago (Zoetmulder 1974, 5; Mulyana 1979, 196; 2005, 84).

Christianity might have existed in the archipelago, albeit insignificantly, as early as the seventh century. However, as a scholar of Indonesia Ismatu Ropi (2000) explains, it was in the early sixteenth century, with the arrival of the Portuguese and the Spanish, that Christianity began to be introduced on a somewhat larger scale. Christianity gained even greater popularity from the end of the sixteenth century alongside the Dutch presence in the archipelago, although it never became a dominant religion (Ropi 2000, 7–10). If missionaries succeeded in converting some people in the archipelago, they did so only in remote areas, such as in North Sumatra, North Sulawesi, Irian, the Moluccas, East Nusa Tenggara, and Central Kalimantan (Suratno 2002, 22; Ropi 2000, 33). This may be related to the fact that the Dutch colonial government prohibited missionaries from entering some areas so as not to provoke any disturbance that would hinder trade. Moreover, some natives resisted the idea of being baptized because converting to Christianity meant serving the interests of the Dutch and losing one's cultural identity (Ropi 2000, 28–29).

The story of when and from where Islam came to Indonesia is an ongoing debate. Nonetheless, scholars believe that teachings of Islam in Indonesia most likely came not directly from Arabs, but by way of (mostly southern) Chinese and/or Indians (possibly Arab-Indians) who traveled to and migrated to Indonesia (Rafferty 1984, 250; Mirpuri 1990, 22; Qurtuby 2003, 37; J. Taylor 2003, 78). That the practice of Islam in Indonesia tends to follow the school of Syafi'iyah, which also existed in India, provides evidence that Islam in Indonesia, at least from the thirteenth to seventeenth centuries, might have come from India/Gujarat (F. Santoso 2002, 48). Moreover, some Islamic stories from Arab lands mostly came from India, specifically south India (Vlekke 1960, 52; Djamaris 1984, 109; Yusuf 1984, 12; J. Taylor 2003, 60). Other scholars credit Muslim-Chinese traders for disseminating Islam broadly throughout the archipelago (Qurtuby 2003, 37).

Indeed, Chinese migration had a long history in Indonesia. Early contacts between Chinese (mostly merchants) and people in Southeast Asia likely began in the early Han period, around the third century CE or possibly earlier, when Chinese merchants traveling by sea began to stop in the archipelago on their way to and from India (Zoetmulder 1974, 5; Irsyam 1985). Although some Chinese migrants had settled in Sriwijaya (a kingdom located in Sumatra) at the end of the seventh century CE, historical evidence shows us that the first permanent settlement of Chinese traders on the north coast of Java dates to the thirteenth century CE (Qurtuby 2003, 73). The number of Chinese settling in Java grew larger at the end of the thirteenth century when the defeated armies of Khubilai Khan settled there (Rafferty 1984, 247–250). In the fifteenth century some Chinese began to settle in Java and interactions between Java and China became more frequent (Qurtuby 2003, 37). It was not until the nineteenth century, however, that large-scale migration from China (mostly Hokkien, Cantonese, Hakka, and Teochiu speakers coming from Fujian and Guangdong provinces of southern China) occurred (Sidel 2006, 19–20). The size of this migration may be related to the fact that the Opium Wars (1839–1842, 1856–1860) had destroyed the economy of those provinces (Irsyam 1985).

Arabs also played an important role in the dissemination of Islam. There are several theories of when Arabs might have first set foot on the archipelago. Some scholars use the dissemination of Islam to theorize that Arabs had begun to migrate to the archipelago in the seventh century (Shahab 1975, 32). However, this forecloses the possibility that Arabs might have come to the archipelago prior to the coming of Islam to seventh-century Arabia. What we do know is that during the twelfth century there were a few Arabs recorded as living in the archipelago who came directly from Arab lands (Vlekke 1960, 52). In addition to these Arabs, there were also "culturally Indian Arabs"—Arabs who had settled in India before coming to Indonesia (Mandal 1994, 17). Large-scale migration from Hadramaut in the southern Arabian Peninsula, where most Arabs in Indonesia had come from, began only in the nineteenth century (Shahab 1975, 36; Mandal 1994, 1, 13).

Buddhist and Hindu practices that were dominant before the coming of Islam also shape the particularities of Islam in Indonesia. In the sixteenth century, for example, Muslims in the archipelago continued to practice Buddhist mystic rituals while giving these practices Arabic names. Kings that were once referred to as "Raja" (a Hindu term) became "Sultans" (a Muslim term) (Geertz 1960, 125). This practice of imbuing rituals of Islam with pre-Islamic traditions still exists in contemporary Indonesia. Javanese traditional rituals such as *sekaten* or *selametan*, for example, are carried out in celebrating Islamic holidays such as *Maulid Nabi Muhammad* (Hadi 2002, 119). Eating diamond-shaped rice (*ketupat*) on the holiday of Eid that is common in present-day Indonesia is actually a practice adapted from the Javanese Hindu tradition (Hadi 2002, 120–121). Indeed, as anthropologist Clifford Geertz pointed out in *Religion of Java*,[1] it was "*abangan*,"[2] (syncretizing "indigenous animism" and "Hindu-Buddhist traditions" in the practice of Islam)[3] that people practiced the most, at least until the 1990s; only one-third of Muslims, at the most, are orthodox or *santri*[4] Muslims (Eliraz 2004, 74).

The second factor that contributes to the particularity of Islam in Indonesia is the influence of neo-modernism from Egypt. Islamic modernism began to be introduced in Indonesia at the end of the nineteenth century, although it's grown rapidly only since the 1970s (Eliraz 2004, 21–23). It was Muhammadiyah, one of two mainstream Islamic organizations[5] in Indonesia, that helped spread Islamic modernism in Indonesia (Mulkhan 2002, 216; Eliraz 2004, 24). This Islamic modernism explains why Indonesian women can participate in education and employment (Eliraz 2004, 21–22). It is important to remember, however, that commitments and practices of Islam in Indonesia differ across regions. For example, people in Sumatra are often regarded as more "radical and fundamentalist," adhering to Islamic *fiqh* (jurisprudence), than people in Java who tend to be more "sufistist" (Mulkhan 2002, 205).

Although Indonesia is the largest Muslim country in the world, Indonesia is not an Islamic state. There were indeed attempts to turn Indonesia into an Islamic rather than a nationalist state in the 1920s and again during the years directly following Indonesia's independence; these attempts, however, failed (Eliraz 2004, 14). Consequently, in Indonesia, laws are not based on Islam and there is a separation between religion and the state (in theory). If Islam influences the Indonesian constitution it is only as far as the concept of monotheism (F. Santoso 2002, 54).

Adding to these already rich cultures was the presence of Europeans. The first Europeans to arrive in the Indies, as had been the case with Chinese and Arab migrants, were mostly males. Although some European women had come to the Dutch East Indies in the 1620s to create a "Dutch settlement" (Locher-Scholten 1992, 265) they encountered various problems and diseases, and female migration was first discouraged, and later even prohibited (except for the wives of higher colonial officers) (Soekiman 2000, 8). European men were then encouraged to keep concubines (*nyai*) (Stoler 2002, 47). The East Indies Company benefited from this arrangement; by encouraging their Dutch male employees to make use of free domestic and sexual services from Asian women, and not have to support a European family, it was possible to keep the European officials' salaries low. These practices also avoided the emergence of "poor white" people, whose very existence might have posed a threat to European white superiority (Stoler 1995, 2002, 48).

However, this concubinage system complicated the meanings of race and racial hierarchies in Indonesia: "Indo" children (children born of sexual unions between Dutch men and native women) could be legally classified as "European" if the European father legally acknowledged the child. This undoubtedly obscured the boundaries between the colonizer and colonized (Stoler 1989). Indeed, Indo women became desirable marriage partners for European men in the colonial Indies (J. Taylor 1992, 255). In later years, and arguably even in today's Indonesia, some Indo women came to represent the epitome of beauty and dominated Indonesian women's magazines. And from the seventeenth to nineteenth centuries, Indo women, along with native concubines, played a crucial role as "mediators," introducing the language of Malay and creole Portuguese commonly spoken at that time, to their European partners (J. Taylor 1992, 255; Locher-Scholten 1992, 266). Of course, in some cases, particularly in the case of those *nyai* who came from relatively poorer Javanese families, such as most *nyai* in Deli (Sumatra), they may not have been able to function as mediators as fully as other *nyai* because they lacked the knowledge and cultural capital to do so (Locher-Scholten 1992, 272–274).

With the opening of the Suez Canal in 1869, this dynamic of interracial relationships in the Indies began to shift with more possibilities for Dutch women to arrive in the Indies with their male counterparts (Soekiman 2000, 8; Lohanda 2002, 8). After the mid-nineteenth century, more European women were allowed to migrate to the archipelago (Stoler 2002, 47).[6] Based on data from 1880, there were 481 European, 620 Chinese, and 830 Arab women migrants for every 1,000 male migrants coming from Europe, China, and Arab lands respectively. By 1930, the number of European women migrants had increased significantly: for every 1,000 European male migrants, there were 884 European women migrants (Riyanto 2000, 41). The number for Chinese and Arab women migrants, however, did not change significantly: for every 1,000 male migrants coming from China and Arab lands, there were 646 Chinese and 841 Arab women migrants (Riyanto 2000, 41). With more European women coming to the archipelago, concubinage began to be represented as less desirable and European men were discouraged from keeping *nyais* (Locher-Scholten 2000, 19; Stoler 2002, 48).

What had not changed drastically in the Indies was how skin color continued to distinguish social categories. During the late ninth and early tenth century in precolonial Java, ideals of beauty highly valued light skin complexion. Throughout the seventeenth and eighteenth centuries, European testimonies stereotyped dark-skinned natives in the Indies as "lazy," "ignorant," and "promiscuous" (Raben 1996, 271, 287). Throughout the colonial period, light-skinned or white-skinned complexion signified higher status. This was reflected in one Indo woman's memoir that narrated how, during her childhood in the colonial Indies, students and teachers valued most highly white and fair-skinned European students at schools (van der Veur 1969, 71). As such, colonialism merely reinforced the pre-existing notion of light-skinned people having higher status (J. Taylor 1992, 256). Paradoxically, in colonial society, as obvious as skin color's importance was, historian Remco Raben has pointed out that "social segmentation did not entirely follow colour lines"; Europeans and "natives" at that time had the tendency to mix and intermarry (1996, 287). And in the postcolonial period, while Westerners are culturally looked up to because of their perceived "superior civilization, high technology and modernity," the Chinese are considered "culturally unattractive" (Heryanto 1999, 161). Although it is evident that in Indonesia race and ethnicity intersect with class and status, a long history of interracial relationships and, in the case of the Chinese, prejudice, complicates their meanings.

Indeed, as political scientist John Sidel pointed out, Dutch colonial policies produced a distinct ethnic Chinese capitalist class that is rendered a "pariah capitalist class," occupying an "outsider" (ethnic) position in Indonesia (2006, 19, 24, 27). The corollary of such a pariah capitalist class whose members did not have access to political or state power was the creation of a "political class" whose members were recruited through educational and religious institutions. Sidel argued that the "matrix of class relations" in today's Indonesia was shaped primarily during and after the colonial era (2006, 18, 36, 42).

What was different during the colonial period, however, was the ways in which skin color was articulated through and conflated with racial discourses. At least that seems to have been the attempt. In a history tracing the development of race or race-consciousness in the Indies, the nineteenth-century period is significant because it was during this period that the Dutch colonial administration carried out various racial projects (Coté 2001, 116; Colombijn 2000, 46). It certainly was during this nineteenth-century period that "white" became a "racial color" category entitling "whites" access to social and economic privileges in everyday lives (Locher-Scholten 2000, 13).

In the Indonesian context, the racial projects that were carried out include the "pass and quarter" system, the cultivation system, the establishment of a legal system, and the installment of a Caucasian white beauty ideal. The pass and quarter system, according to historian Sumit Mandal, allowed for the emergence of race by requiring natives and "Foreign Orientals" to carry "passes" for travel (1816–1910); the "quarter" system (1866–1910), by regulating "obligatory residential zones," particularly for "Foreign Orientals" (1994, 57–60, 84), raised the question of who would be counted as native, who as Foreign Oriental. The need to classify oneself racially therefore became important for defining where and how people would live and travel. In this sense, racial categories are mapped, quite literally, onto processes of racial formation.

Still another racial project made racial differences in the Indies more visible: the *Sistem Tanam Paksa/Cultuurstelsel* (Forced Cultivation System) enacted in 1830 (Gouda 1995, 24). The Dutch enriched themselves and impoverished natives, expropriating native land and labor, henceforth requiring natives to pay rent plus two-fifths of their agricultural products. Under this system, the Dutch also took over sugar plantations and factories, managing if not owning these factories (Knight 2000, xvi). The colonial government ended the Cultivation System in 1870, and its new Agrarian Law, which allowed private capital ownership, encouraged investors primarily from the United States and Europe (Riyanto 2000, 31). Dutch, Belgian, and French companies were given concessions for palm oil in East Sumatra and Aceh, for example, and massive investment from the United States and England, was counterbalanced by concessions to Japanese who were allowed to invest in Indonesia in the period 1916 to 1924 (Post 1994, 303; Ismail 1996, 240). In the early 1930s, when tariffs and quota protection were put into place, multinational companies, including Unilever, British American Tobacco (BAT), Bata, and Goodyear, began to open factories in Indonesia (Wie 1996, 326). It was during this time when people in the Indies, particularly working-class people, began to be introduced to "money" as an exchange system (Riyanto 2000, 32).

Moreover, racial project was also manifested in the field of law. In 1854, two separate legal codes were established to provide different laws (civil, commerce, civil procedure, criminal procedure) for Europeans and non-Europeans. Because individuals could not be tried under European law if they were not European, the need to be able to identify and be identified as a European became significant; yet, because in the Indies, "European" in its legal sense did not simply refer to people originally from Europe, many people attempted to be classified as Europeans. For example, legally acknowledged daughters of a European father and a non-European woman who then married to a European male would demand and usually be granted European equivalence (Gouda 1995, 163). It is true that in these cases, their access to Europeanness was still tied to their connection to European males, yet, when Japanese people living in the Indies received the right to have "European equivalence," the notion of Europeanness lost its "racial connotation[s]" (Fasseur 1997, 37–40). Indeed, as Ann Stoler pointed out, by the beginning of the twentieth century, not only Japanese, but also "Jews, Arabs, Armenians, Filipinos, naturalized Javanese, Sundanese wives of Dutch-born bureaucrats, recognized children of mixed marriages, and Christian Africans" could legally be considered European as long as they were Christian, fluent in Dutch, Dutch-educated, "demonstrate[d] suitability for European society," or married to or adopted by Europeans (2002, 39). It needs to be emphasized, though, that this European equivalence was a legal category and did not necessarily bring about significant changes in the everyday lives of most people in the Indies (Fasseur 1997, 40–41). This actually further complicated the process of establishing a white racial category that relied on skin color as one of its signifiers. In other words, attempts to conflate skin color and race in practice through these racial projects might not be so straightforward as it might seem as "policies." To further complicate the reality of such racial projects, in 1920, approximately 90 percent of people categorized as "Europeans" were "Indo-Europeans" (Bashford and Levine 2010, 353).

Nonetheless, one of the ramifications of this "suitability for European society" policy was that "performing" Europeanness then became more and more important in the Indies. One certainly had to perform Europeanness if he or she were to claim membership in elite colonial society (Protschky 2008, 348). Moreover, the increasing presence of Dutch women in the Indies around this time further reinforced the need to perform Europeanness to mark the boundaries between the colonized and the colonizer—a boundary that was loosely guarded and frequently traversed by way of concubinage and interracial marriage prior to Dutch women's arrival in the Indies.

What constituted performing Europeanness was unclear, however. Signifiers for Europeanness had to be aggressively constructed and outwardly displayed. Dutch women in particular were encouraged to surround themselves and their family with the cultural artifacts of "being European" (Stoler 1989, 640). To do so, Dutch women had to learn the proper commodities to consume and the proper way to behave from colonial manuals (Schulte 1997, 26). If these women had to learn about European notions of middle-class respectability and "colonial propriety" prior to coming to the Indies it is because they bore the burden of upholding "white prestige" (Stoler 1989, 648, 652). However, because performing Europeanness provided one's access to membership in the elite group, European commodities were not only consumed by Europeans to guard their prestige as the colonizer but also as a form of cultural capital for Indos (mixed race people), Chinese, and new native *priyayis* (Javanese bureaucrats and aristocrats) who deployed European culture to advance their career, prestige, and social and political status (Onghokham 1997, 177–179; Soekiman 2000, 36).

It is worth clarifying here that *priyayi* is a concept that clearly shows the intersection of class, status, religion, and to some extent ethnicity—Chinese were not constructed as *priyayi*. Aristocratic and bureaucratic *priyayi*, like *abangan*, were/are non-orthodox Muslims. I'd like to turn to Geertz here who has provided us with a useful understanding of these concepts. He argues that what sets *abangan* apart from *priyayi* was their class position: *abangan* were Java's peasantry, the *priyayi* "its gentry"—most of these *priyayi* were not "landed gentry" or "baronial landlords," however. Particularly under Dutch colonial rule, *priyayi* was often used to refer to "bureaucrats, clerks, and teachers—white-collar nobles" (1973, 229). They were the ones benefiting from Dutch colonial education and working for Dutch companies. *Priyayi* were Western-educated Javanese with Dutch manners and values and usually spoke Dutch instead of Javanese.[7] As such, they were "pro-government" and "pro-status quo" (Sutherland 1979, 28). Their roles were particularly significant during the *Tanam Paksa* (Cultivation System)[8] period, 1830–1870, in controlling the natives and collecting taxes on behalf of the Dutch colonial government (Riyanto 2000, 30).

Priyayi often claimed that they were descendants of the "semi-mythical kings of precolonial Java," "rulers of ancient Java," or "early Islamic Saints," and bore aristocratic titles such as R.M. (Raden Mas) or, for a wife, R.A. (Raden Ayu) (Geertz 1973, 229; Sutherland 1979, 5). These *priyayi*, however, usually had *selir* (subsequent wives or mistresses who were taken to live in the palace) who might include women of Chinese, Arab, or Indo descent.

Priyayi sometimes had sumptuous lifestyles. Europeans in the Indies, at least in the eighteenth and nineteenth centuries, often modeled their "houses, food, clothes, language, wives and entertainments" after these *priyayi* (Sutherland 1979, 36). By the end of the nineteenth century, however, with the first publications of fiction highlighting suffering caused by colonialism, it appears that sumptuous living was no longer admired (Sutherland 1979, 42). Nonetheless, the emphasis on and continuing desire for aristocrat or royal culture can be seen in post-Independence Indonesia with marriage ceremonies that reenact royal weddings and brides and grooms who dress as princesses and princes (Geertz 1973, 57). In spite of their aristocratic status and lifestyle, *priyayi* did not have access to controlling the colonial economy. It was the colonial administration, unsurprisingly, who regulated the economy and capital investments (Zed 1996, 251–252).

Worth mentioning here is the fact that "Dutch culture" was brought to the Indies not only by Dutch people but also by native (particularly Javanese) scholars who studied in the Netherlands (Soekiman 2000, 36). This further added to the complexity of the flow of culture between the Netherlands and the Indies. Because people from various backgrounds used European commodities as a form of cultural capital, material or cultural adeptness to European culture was no longer sufficient to claim suitability for European society. People also needed to show that they had the "psychological dispositions" of "Europeans," achievable through training in "European morals and ideas" (Stoler 1996, 73–74).

It is then that what I call "colonial emotionology" became an important affective apparatus in marking one's identity—an identity that was regulated and expressed through emotions. Historians Carol Stearns and Peter Stearns define emotionology as "the attitudes or standards that a society, or a definable group within a society, maintains toward basic emotions and their appropriate expression: ways that institutions reflect and encourage these attitudes in human conduct" (Stearns and Stearns 1985, 813). Emotionology could also be understood as "ideologically-permitted emotions" (Locher-Scholten 2000, 97). Some people are ideologically permitted to express certain emotions whereas some others are not because the expressions of these emotions function to naturalize social differences and serve the purpose of the ruling elites. As feminist philosopher Alison Jaggar (1989) argues through her notion of "emotional hegemony," gendered discourse of emotions functions to serve the interests of the male ruling elites. Building on these concepts, I define "colonial emotionology" as the ways in which ideologically permitted emotions as an articulation of the self serve the interests of the colonial empire. Emotionology thus does the work of producing a sense of "*felt* belonging"—an identity that works through the body, its senses, and the mind ("the intelligible") (Ahmed and Stacey 2000, 16). This sense of felt belonging reflects how subjectivity formation is an effect of an ideology of emotions. Pointing out the formation of affectively produced subjectivity is important because as cultural studies scholars Jennifer Harding and Deidre Pribram argue, "the subject who feels is critical to the circulation of power, the establishment of social relations, and the construction of discursive and institutional formations" (2004, 879).

According to "colonial emotionology" in the Dutch East Indies, Dutch women were discouraged from showing their emotions. They also had to withhold their emotions to distinguish themselves as the respectable colonial female employer, from their native servants. Thus colonialism hinged, in part, on Dutch women's ability to display signs of white prestige not only through material and cultural signifiers but also through their emotional and psychological dispositions, governed by "colonial emotionology." Historian Elsbeth Locher-Scholten studied the manuals written for white women in the Indies and showed that white women were advised to react in "a wise and restrained manner," and when dealing with their servants they had to be "calm, self-possessed, never angry, but always resolute and superior" (2000, 96–97). Hence to remain superior, they had to refrain from being angry or using harsh scolding. This is so because anger, particularly for white women, was an inappropriate emotion that could lower white prestige; indeed, "prestige was the reason behind proper and restrained behaviour" (Locher-Scholten 2000, 97). The relationship between emotion and class can also be observed in Javanese communities as there is the need to preserve a certain flatness of affect among upper-class Javanese/*priyayi* (Geertz 1960, 240). Moreover, in the Old Javanese version of *Ramayana*, it was stated that "control of the senses is the most beloved wife [of a king]" (*Ramayana* 628). This highlights once again the intricate relationship between social expressions of emotion and class status.

I argue that white prestige was what grounded "colonial emotionology." In this sense, affect functions as a technology of surveillance and as an apparatus of power that disciplines white women's bodies. This gendered representation of white women as the calm (restraint in displaying emotions) and delicate face of beauty could easily be seen in women's magazines around this period.

Women's Magazines and European White Beauty

At the beginning of the twentieth century, there occurred a shift in Dutch colonial politics marked by the implementation of a so-called ethical policy in 1901. This policy, which basically attempted to cope with some of the negative effects of colonialism, actually allowed for the development of an early nationalist movement (Rutherford 1998, 258; Coté 2001, 128). For example, in 1908 *Budi Utomo*, an organization for bettering natives' education, was founded. *Sarekat*

Islam, the Islamic Association, was established around 1912 (Scholte 1995, 196). The ethical policy brought changes particularly in the realm of education, providing limited access to education, hence literacy, for some privileged natives. However, prior to the implementation of the ethical policy, schools for natives began to emerge in the late nineteenth century (Riyanto 2000, 41). At that time, schools were divided into four categories: European curriculum schooling for Europeans; Dutch language schooling for native elites; local language schooling for some other natives; and traditional schooling such as *pesantren* (Islamic schools) for other natives (Riyanto 2000, 42). In addition to these schools there were also schools for Chinese such as *Hollands-Chineesche* (Locher-Scholten 2000, 19). Although girls were not legally barred from getting a basic education, they were not allowed to attend advanced schooling (J. Taylor 2003, 289). Only a small number of aristocratic girls had access to education (Riyanto 2000, 41). In 1898, for example, there were only 2,891 girls in school in the entire East Indies (Kartini 2002, 13). Nonetheless, access to education was crucial in initiating the process of modernity for native women in general at that time. These educated women, including Raden Ayu (aristocratic title) Kartini—Indonesia's early "feminist"—then began to demand and establish schools for girls, advocate monogamy, and participate in larger nationalist struggles. By 1930, 10 percent of men in Java and Madura could read, but only 1.5 percent of women could read and write either Dutch or Indonesian.[9] Only 34,000 native women, compared to 102,000 men living in Java, could write Dutch (Locher-Scholten 2000, 19).

It was these (mostly male) educated natives who then contributed to the development of various newspapers,[10] even women's periodicals, in their attempts to "imagine" a nation. As Southeast Asian specialist Benedict Anderson pointed out in his book *Imagined Communities*, the technology of print-capitalism that allows for (re)production and dissemination of newspapers provided the material basis for the emergence of national consciousness and the ways in which community is imagined. This means that at this particular moment in history, the end of the nineteenth and the early twentieth centuries, when early nationalists began to formulate their national identities, writers and newspapers played a significant role.

Sociologist Tamrin Amal Tomagola, in his dissertation "Indonesian Women's Magazines as an Ideological Medium," traces the history of women's magazines in Indonesia back to 1906 when a Chinese woman, Liem Titie Nio, created a "special women's section" in a Malay-language newspaper (1990, 49). That women's newspapers began as "special sections" was also true in the case of Dutch-language newspapers such as *Bataviaasch Nieuwsblad* (1885–1935), *De Locomotief* (1864–1956), and *Java Bode* (1852–1957) published in the archipelago (Locher-Scholten 2000, 136, 138, 144). At first, these women's magazines mostly discussed "domestic matters," but they then shifted their focus to political issues, a change coinciding with the development of the nationalist movement and the women's movement in particular, beginning in the 1920s (Tomagola 1990, 60).

Periodicals published under colonial rule, not surprisingly, provide ample evidence that Caucasian women were represented as the beauty ideal in the dominant beauty discourse and that beauty and skin products said to whiten one's skin were already being marketed. Here, I explicitly say "dominant" to suggest that there were also competing discourses of women's beauty even at this time. In this first half of the twentieth century, advertisements usually consisted of a few paragraphs of written texts and very minimal, if at all, black and white drawings. Most beauty product ads, however, usually included black and white drawings of Caucasian women accompanied by texts that signify them as the beauty ideal. For example, the caption accompanying the black and white drawing of a Caucasian woman suggested "how the most beautiful women in the world maintain their beauty" by using Palmolive soap (*De Huisvrouw in Indie* 1937). Not only inviting its women readers to use this soap, the ad also reveals and sells the idea that Caucasian women were the beauty ideal. Furthermore, after the boom in American films in the 1920s and 1930s (Locher-Scholten 2000, 135), there were black and white photographic drawings of (white) American movie stars such as Irene Dunne (*De Huisvrouw* 1938), Deanna Durbin (*De Huisvrouw* 1939 and *De Huisvrouw in Nord Sumatra* 1939), Claudette Colbert (*De Huisvrouw in Indie* 1940 and *De Huisvrouw in Nord Sumatra* 1940), and Loretta Young (*De Huisvrouw in Indie* 1941), all advertising Lux beauty soap while reaffirming the Caucasian beauty ideal. Significantly, however, drawings of Caucasian women were found not only in Dutch-language periodicals for Dutch women, such as *De Huisvrouw*, but also in Malay-language periodicals for natives such as *Bintang Hindia*. For example, in an ad for "Roos-perzie" poepoer (beauty mask) in *Bintang Hindia* (1928), the beautiful woman represented was a Caucasian woman.

More than simply selling beauty products, the ads circulating around this time were also selling the idea of white as the desirable skin color, with white skin color being conflated with white race, a racial category representing a particular gendered emotionality of restraint. This was different from the beauty ideal during the late ninth century and early tenth century in precolonial Java, in that the light-skinned women who were considered beautiful at that time were not necessarily whites, let alone members of the Caucasian white race. It was only during the Dutch colonial era that white, as a skin color began to refer to white, meaning Caucasian race—the meanings of white skin color were therefore conflated with the meanings of white race. As can be seen in the ads circulated around this time, products with Caucasian models, ranging from "medicated" skin powder, such as Virgin powder and Ninon powder, to Snow cold cream, usually claimed to make people's skin white (*putih*, which literally means the color of and not necessarily the race of white). In some ads that did not explicitly claim to whiten one's skin, there still appeared a suggestion that these products could make one's complexion "better." In an ad for Pond's, for example, a Caucasian woman whose gaze shies away from the camera is wearing a tiara signifying her aristocratic position, as "Lady Morris." The text that accompanied her image claimed that Pond's improved her complexion (*De Huisvrouw* 1939). Of course, it was understood that an improved complexion would resemble a "lady's." And this notion of "Lady" as a signifier for Caucasian white beauty was particularly important in representing the restrained, lady-like behavior of European white women at the time. This lady-like manner indeed seems to have been the norm in beauty ads. Another ad, for Yardley Lavender, featured a drawing of an aristocratic woman elegantly holding a bottle of the Yardley product with only four fingers as if holding a very fragile product, her pinky finger held apart from the rest of her fingers in a delicate and feminine manner (*De Huisvrouw* 1937). The seemingly exaggerated display of femininity in most of these ads underscores the "colonial emotionology" of acceptable emotional expressions for Caucasian white women. Not only that: this gendered "colonial emotionology" that restrained Caucasian white women's expression of affect functioned as a technology of discipline and surveillance. By being allowed only a limited range of emotions in these ads, Caucasian white women models' bodies are being disciplined by "affect" as its apparatus of power.

Although these ads usually targeted women, there were some whitening ads that also targeted men. For example, an ad for Bedak Dingin Extract (cold cream), published in *Keng Po* (January 6, 1934), specifically stated that this product was useful for men who wanted a smooth, clean, and white face. Interestingly, although the product targeted men, the testimony, which was part of the ad, suggested that it was women who used these products:

> I, signing this letter, R.M. Soedarsono alias Koornen Reclame Toekenaar, live on Manggabesar No. 41A Batavia. I would like to inform you that my wife Soevijah uses cold cream extract from Chun Lim & Co. in Batavia and six days later her black/dark-skinned (*hitam*) face became yellow (*kuning*) and clean. I attest that this cold cream extract of Chun Lim & Co. is indeed incredible and very useful to make one's skin white, as was demonstrated by my wife.

This ad is particularly interesting because first, the one who testifies here is an elite male, signified by R.M., short for Raden Mas, an aristocratic Javanese title.

It therefore positions and uses his distinct social status in colonial society to market its products.

Second, the fact that it was a man who wrote the testimony rather than the woman who actually used the product reveals the gender order of the time when men's voices were not only considered more valuable than women's voices but also men's narratives were needed to validate women's experience. Not only that, but being married to a light-skinned women was considered preferable during that time. A comment made in 1925 suggested that if men could afford it, they preferred to keep their wives at home because they "like[d] pretty hands and a pretty complexion" (Locher-Scholten 2000, 50). Such a comment once again reveals the relationship between high status, class, and light skin color. It also indicates the extent to which complexion was a factor in describing attractive women. Remaining at home, that is out of the sun, would indicate the importance of light skin; and that the injunction against waged or salaried work was strongest for upper-class women would indicate a relationship to economic class. Nonetheless, because the economic condition of most colonized men necessitated that their wives work outside the home, many women did.[11]

Third, R.M. Soedarsono's letter does not seem to differentiate between yellow and white skin color. He even used his wife's skin transformation from black to yellow to support his argument that the cold cream could make one's skin white. Equating white and yellow may simply be carelessness on the part of the advertiser. However, it may also reveal the underlying skin color order at that time: white skin color was conflated with white race and thus only Europeans could be considered "whites." Hence, although both white and yellow were considered light skin colors, white was used to refer to the colonial race and yellow, light-skinned natives.

This notion of "yellow" as the ideal color for natives could also be seen in fiction writing. In a serial story, "Nyai Ratna," published in *Medan Prijaji* in 1909, Tirto Adhi Soerjo, an important Indonesian nationalist described the beautiful Nyai Ratna as "true, not white, only yellow" (Toer 1985, 301). Describing Nyai Ratna as "not white," but "only yellow" reveals the color hierarchy of a time when white was considered the preferred color and yellow the second preferred color. However, it might also be read as the text's refusal to define "native" beauty through the racialized white color defined by the colonizer.

And finally, because in R.M. Soedarsono's letter it was his wife who used this product, it suggests that it was women rather than men who mostly purchased the product. After all, as can be read in a memoir of one Indo woman, it was mostly women who were told to "[b]e careful that you do not tan" so that they could attract white men of good position (van der Veur 1969, 71).

It is evident, therefore, that during Dutch colonization the meanings of skin color shifted in the Indies. I do not, however, suggest that simply by being present, the Dutch shifted the meanings of light skin color within the beauty discourse. Rather, it was their powerful position as the colonizer that framed their encounters with other people in the Indies, allowing them to circulate the idea of Caucasian women as the epitome of beauty within the frame of white race supremacy. This was challenged when Japan managed to replace the Dutch as colonizer in the Indies.

ROUTING WHITENESS: JAPAN AND THE NEW ASIAN WHITE BEAUTY IDEAL (1942–1945)

The Japanese occupation, which began in March 1942, lasted "only" three years and five months. A Japanese presence in the Indies, however, predates the occupation and made a far more significant impact on Indonesian culture than the brief occupation would suggest. A small Japanese community had existed in Batavia (now Jakarta) since the early seventeenth century or possibly earlier (Blussé 1986, 187). Under the Dutch, it is significant to note, the Japanese community occupied a separate and privileged position compared to native Indonesians. Moreover, even before occupying Indonesia, the Japanese, as Asians, had inspired the emergence of a "Javanese political consciousness" by defeating Russia in 1905 (Locher-Scholten 1986, 10). Undoubtedly it was during their occupation when Japan's influence had its most significant impact on Indonesia, reconfiguring even the meanings of skin color.

At the heart of the Japanese occupation were various racial projects that engendered a new racial hierarchy. Within this new racial order, Asians were considered superior (at the top of the hierarchy were Japanese; second were Indonesians, Chinese, Arabs, and Indians), while "non-Asian nationalities," including European and Eurasians who had occupied privileged positions before, now had to occupy the bottom rank (Touwen-Bouwsma 1995, 8, 15–16).

In establishing and maintaining this hierarchy, Japan carried out various policies and projects. For example, Japan set up internment camps to isolate Europeans and Eurasians, although in practice it was Eurasians more than Europeans who ended up in the internment camps. The reason for this may be related to the fact that Japanese culture valued "racial homogeneity" and "racial purity." Consequently, Indos or mixed-blood Eurasians were considered inferior and became the target of punitive measures. One of the ways in which these Eurasians could avoid being punished, however, was by proving that they had at least 50 percent Indonesian ancestry and had adopted an Indonesian lifestyle. Hence, it was during this occupation that Eurasians, who had previously covered up their Indonesian origins, now claimed their Indonesian background and were even encouraged to abandon their racial ties to their European ancestors (Touwen-Bouwsma 1995, 10, 15).

The Japanese also carried out large-scale propaganda to instill the notion of Asian racial superiority, in part to convince Indonesians that they too had a stake in the Japanese war. (Should Indonesians assist Japan in winning the war, they would then be liberated under the "Greater East Asian Co-prosperity Sphere" [*Kemakmuran Bersama Asia Timur Raya*]). In disseminating this propaganda, Japan recruited several highly visible nationalists including Soekarno, who later became Indonesia's first president. Clearly, in collaborating with the Japanese, Soekarno would have thought that he could use Japan's resources in the interest of the nationalist movement (Locher-Scholten 1986, 20–21). Additionally, in assuring that their propaganda reached all walks of life, the Japanese commissioned several artists to compose pro-Japanese/pro-Asian songs, plays, dances, and speeches that were performed live or disseminated via radio, film, and magazines (Kurasawa 1990, 487–490). Some examples of their propaganda include a well-known wayang puppet shadow play that narrated a story of how Pandawa (the heroes in the *Mahabharata*), representing Indonesia, were being helped by the Sun God, representing the Japanese, in winning the war. Another example was a western Javanese (Sundanese) traditional dance performance called "Defeating America/England Dance" (*Tari Meruntuhkan Amerika/Inggris*) that propagated Asian superiority over Europeans (Yuliati et al. 2002, 6).

Reading through various magazines and newspapers published during the Japanese occupation, I found that Indonesians themselves participated in propagating the idea that Asians and their values were better than Western values. In *Almanak Asia Raya*, for example, an Indonesian male nationalist, Soewandhie, wrote how Indonesians, who had suffered under the colonial rule of the white-skinned nation (*bangsa kulit putih*), need to happily embrace the change brought about by Japanese presence in the Indies (*Almanak Asia Raya* 1943, 65). In further promoting Asian values, he then invoked everything Asian, such as "Indian philosophy," "Persian literature," and "Chinese ethics" (*Almanak Asia Raya* 1943, 68). In another and more subtle article, published in *Djawa Baroe*, and written by one of Indonesia's most well-known women journalists, H. Diah, Diah wrote that after having lived for several years in the United States and in Japan, she became aware of how "Nippon" women were different from American women. Nippon women's style and attitude were "attractive" because they were *jelita* (literally "beautiful"). American women, she wrote, were "aggressive" or "daring" (*menantang*) (*Djawa Baroe* 8). She ended the article by pointing out that "East is East and West is West" (*Djawa Baroe* 9) and that the two could never meet, suggesting however implicitly that both Eastern countries, Indonesia and Japan, could work together while Indonesia and a Western country such as the United States could not. What is lurking behind these articles are sentiments and feelings toward certain groups. In other words, these articles did the work of circulating certain feelings about certain people thus creating the "felt belonging" identity.

This racial project, representing Asians as superior to Europeans, was also evident in women's beauty discourses. In publications such as *Djawa Baroe* and *Almanak Asia Raya*, there were obvious attempts to reconstruct an ideal women's beauty. If periodicals prior to the Japanese occupation represented Caucasian women as the epitome of beauty, these Malay-language periodicals, established for the purpose of disseminating Japanese propaganda, represented Japanese and Indonesian women as the beautiful ones. *Djawa Baroe*, for example, carried columns such as "Nippon Girls" (*Putri Nippon*), "Nippon Movie Stars" (*Bintang Film Nippon*), and "Beautiful Indonesian Girls" (*Putri Indonesia Yang Cantik Molek*), where beautiful Japanese and Indonesian women were praised for their beauty. In these columns, the captions accompanying pictures of Japanese movie stars, who all wore kimonos, usually mentioned that these women were "beautiful" (*cantik*) and "have elegant manners" (*lemah lembut budi bahasanya*) (*Djawa Baroe* 1943). In the "Beautiful Indonesian Girls" column, there were pictures of Indonesian women, mostly from Java, but also from Minahasa (Sulawesi) and Minangkabau (Sumatra). Indonesian women, like the Japanese ones, wore traditional clothing and were all relatively light skinned. In noting the consistency of traditional clothing in these pictures, I agree with historian Anton Lucas (1997, 60) who points out that in reconstructing a new Asian beauty ideal, Japan had to revive the image of a traditional Asian beauty ideal to counter the modern European woman.

It even seems that traditional clothing was the only signifier that differentiated these Asian women from European women. Lucas points out that although Japan attempted to promote an ideal of Asian beauty, the images of these beautiful women seem to be "Western" if not "Western-influenced" and were "little different from Western images" (Lucas 1997, 67, 78). For example, in *Djawa Baroe*, there was an advertisement for *Lotos* powder. In this ad, a woman wears traditional clothing, a *kebaya*, but her facial features and skin color seem to suggest that she is European or Eurasian. In another magazine, *Soeara Asia*, there was an ad for "as white as pearls" toothpaste, in which the woman also seems to be of European descent. Another ad in the same periodical, for lipstick, portrays a woman, wearing traditional *kebaya*, with European facial features. Additionally, in a column that contains pictures of radio and theater stars, Eurasian women such as Fifi Young and Sally Young were most often represented (*Soeara Asia* 1943). All of this suggests that although, in theory, Japanese could claim success in reconstructing a new Asian beauty ideal superior to Western beauty, in practice, the Asian women, even when wearing traditional Asian clothing, did not look that much different from Western women.

Why was this attempt to reconstruct an ideal Asian beauty successful in theory but a failure in practice? This contradiction may be explained by two factors. First, although it was Asian beauty that was promoted, it was still white or light skin that was considered desirable. Certainly a distinction needs to be made here: this "white" skin was not necessarily European white. Here, skin color was dissociated from race. Nonetheless, while it was possible to make the distinction in theory, in practice it was rather difficult because the desirable color was still white. After all, when white skin color does not really exist, how can one differentiate one white skin from another? This inability to articulate the "new" color that the Japanese brought to the Indies was metaphorically represented by a 1944 ad for Club powder in *Djawa Baroe*. In this ad, a very light-skinned Japanese woman is applying a powder puff to her cheek as if she were putting powder on her face. The caption reads, "when women try it once, they will understand that this powder is really good, smells nice, has a really *new color* (*warnanya baru sekali*) and makes many people *happy*" (emphasis mine). What is intriguing here is that it wasn't clear what this "new color" was. Although this ad could simply be read as advertising a new line of color, when other ads during this period such as for Virgin powder or Ajer Daffodil (the ones without Japanese women models) could still name and claim to make one's skin white, this particular Japanese ad that did not specify what this new color was reveals the tension in articulating and naming a new color. Moreover, this emphasis on attaining happiness through consumption of a new color underscores the ways in which the ad relies on the working of emotions as "techniques of discipline that help shape what we do and who we are" (Harding and Pribram quoted in Harding and Pribram 2004, 879). Happiness therefore becomes an affective apparatus that disciplines the body and even dictates its color. Moreover, through these beauty ads, people's subjectivity was affectively interpellated—ads call our subjectivity into being through the feelings they attempt to evoke. Emotions thus function as an apparatus of power when we feel compelled to do what the ads persuade us to do because we see it as a way to make us feel good, or whatever feeling the advertised commodity promises.

The second factor that helps explain the failure of reconstructing an ideal Asian beauty in practice relates to Japanese claims to whiteness, their ambivalent relationship to whiteness, and their being considered honorary Europeans. For the Japanese, who historically were considered "honorary Europeans" and in the Indies had been granted "European equivalence," whiteness, let alone white skin, was not considered the sole possession of Europeans. Japanese and

Chinese societies indeed had preferred the color white and referred to themselves as "whites." Note, however, that their considering themselves whites referred to the whiteness of their skin color and not race.

Even prior to contacts with Europeans or Africans, Japanese people already considered white skin beautiful and black skin ugly. For the Japanese, white skin color had been considered beautiful even prior to its conflation with race. In constructing the history of skin color in Japan, anthropologist Hiroshi Wagatsuma pointed out that an old Japanese proverb affirms that "'white skin makes up for seven defects'; a woman's light skin causes one to overlook the absence of other desired physical features" (1967, 407). During the Nara period (710–793), aristocratic women used white powder to whiten their face. From the eighth to the twelfth century, white was the beauty ideal in literature; it was also a marker of upper-class women because these women did not have to work outside and get their skin tanned. In the seventeenth century, white continued to be the beauty ideal even as the ideal shape of beauty shifted from voluptuous to slim women (Wagatsuma 1967, 407–409).

In the Japanese context, this conflation between white skin color and Western whiteness of race could be traced to the late nineteenth century, particularly during the Meiji period (1868–1912), when the Japanese came to consider Europeans their "model to emulate" (Creighton 1997, 216). Preference for white skin in Japan, which was traditionally not about European white skin, then became integrated with European whiteness (Bonnett 2002, 92). An interesting development occurred in the 1920s, when the Japanese began to position Caucasian white skin color as "whiter" than Japanese white skin color, but then a shift occurred in the mid-1930s when the ultra-nationalist government put an end to representation of the Western world as superior (Wagatsuma 1967, 416, 435). Nonetheless, after Japanese notions of skin color had been so infused with a Western notion of white skin, it became rather difficult to articulate a new white Asian beauty ideal that was completely separated from Caucasian whiteness.

Interestingly, Japan was more successful in articulating a notion of distinctive Japanese whiteness, while still admiring Caucasian whiteness in the postwar period and even more so in contemporary Japan. Since the postwar era, "mainstream" Japan has gained a high level of economic achievement and privilege and may have entered what anthropologist Millie Creighton referred to as "the *symbolic space* of 'white,' the cognitive space of prominence and ascendancy" and even feel that they are better than Westerners (1997, 220, 221). Indeed, as Mikiko Ashikari (2005) argues in "Cultivating Japanese Whiteness," skin-lightening products are popular in contemporary Japan because Japanese women desire a Japanese whiteness that is considered better than Caucasian whiteness—Caucasian white skin color is considered "'ugly' in texture and quality" (Wagatsuma

1967, 435). Such a claim is only possible when the concept of skin color is understood as something that is divorced from race: a person can have white skin color without being a member of Caucasian white race.

CONCLUSION: WHY WHITE AFTER ALL?

These constructions of whiteness from European to Japanese whiteness highlight the ways in which race is conflated with, and then dissociated from, skin color. This construction is unlike in the United States where skin color functions as a signifier for race. One may wonder, however, why there is such persistence in claiming the "self" (Caucasian or Japanese) as embodying whiteness. Might it be related to the fact that the color of white has good connotative meanings? Psychologist John Williams, writing within a Western context, has suggested that people transfer the connotative meanings of white as "good" to the white-coded race and the meanings of black as "bad" to the black-coded race (1997, 238). Geographer Yi Fu Tuan also acknowledges that in Western and non-Western cultures, while white has some negative connotations, it mostly holds positive meanings such as "light, hope, joy, and purity" while black has negative meanings (1974/1990, 25). Might people consequently prefer to understand themselves to be white of whatever race or nation in order to be considered "good"? Indeed, during the pre–Civil War period in the United States people may have assigned themselves the category of white because of its connotative meanings as "not slaves" rather than simply to use it as an "accurate term to describe [their] skin color" (Dyer 1997, 50). Because whiteness is indeed an ambiguous and arbitrary construction, it allows for the possibility to claim whiteness even if one does not have "white" skin color. After all, who literally has white skin color?

It is precisely this ambiguity that gives whiteness its strength. Race scholar Richard Dyer argues,

> white as skin colour is just as unstable, unbounded a category as white as a hue, and therein lies its strength. It enables whiteness to be presented as an apparently attainable, flexible, varied category, while setting up an always movable criterion of inclusion, the ascribed whiteness of your skin. (1997, 57)

This imagined possibility of attaining whiteness allows people of various nations to claim their own and give new meanings to whiteness. Nonetheless, as it is whiteness that is being claimed, it merely strengthens rather than challenges whiteness as the dominant color across nations.

If claiming whiteness actually strengthens the position of whiteness in a global racial hierarchy, why construct an ideal beauty that is represented by white or light-skinned women? The answer seems to lie within the argument that modernity is often conflated with Western/whiteness. As social geographer Alastair Bonnett points out, the "white" race actually benefits from the conflation Western/whiteness/modernity because to achieve modernity one needs to adopt "racial whiteness." In the specific Venezuelan case that Bonnett discusses, he points out that to achieve "national advancement" requires that the nation take the "route towards whiteness" (2002, 69–70, 77). Certainly, there is a danger in propagating whiteness, albeit an Asian one, as a superior color. That is, because it is whiteness that is being claimed, it merely strengthens rather than challenges whiteness as the dominant color across nations.

A second answer to the question "why conflate beauty and whiteness" may relate to the fact that it is white that is internationally recognized as having a currency within a global context. Even Japan adopts whiteness to validate its power over other Asian nations (Bonnett 2002, 94). What this means is that although it is possible to represent darker-skinned women as the beauty standard, because national identity is about representing the self not only to its citizens but also to other nations, these dark-skinned women may not be internationally recognized as beautiful. This actually exposes how the construction of light-skinned women as beautiful cannot be guarded by only one nation. Even the United States, however powerful it may be, cannot alone impose this idea. Particularly because people and objects move across nations, there needs to be some kind of reinforcement not only in the country of departure but also in the country of destination. In other words, structures of power can be maintained across different localities because these different locations support and validate each other's power structure.

This chapter clearly demonstrates that white subjectivity in colonial Indonesia is not a mere narrative of European whiteness. The Japanese colonizer challenged the European white beauty ideal by offering their own version of an Asian white beauty ideal. However, although Asian was constructed as the preferred race, white remained the preferred color, with dark skin configured as undesirable. Nonetheless, this notion that Europeans are not the sole possessor of whiteness is important for it led to and provided the theoretical and psychological space for the construction of the "Indonesian whiteness" in the postcolonial period.

3 | Indonesian White Beauty

Spatializing Race and
Racializing Spatial Tropes

"Where are you from?" a fellow scholar politely asked me. A bit of small talk seemed appropriate: we were shoving our belongings into the lockers of KITLV library in Leiden, the Netherlands. It was the summer of 2006. I was then a graduate student doing research for my dissertation. "Well, I live in Canada, but I go to school in the United States; this summer, I am staying with my sister in France. So, where should I say I am from?" I playfully threw the question right back at him, purposefully omitting "Indonesia" in my answer to subtly hint at and expose the complexity and racial undertone of his question, although I then realized that I sounded pretentious in the process.

"But where are you from, *originally*?" he then asked. I smiled, knowing that that question was coming: my "race" could not be traced back to these places. "Indonesia," I finally said with the answer I thought would satisfy his curiosity. Yet, he refused to let that be my final answer and asked another question, "But you didn't grow up in Indonesia, did you? Your accent, it's not Indonesian." This time it was my accent that seemed to betray my race, my face, and my "place of origin." "I was born and raised in Indonesia. I don't know how I got this accent. Perhaps I watch too much American television," I jovially answered before excusing myself—"Nice meeting you." I gently closed my locker door and courteously ended the small talk.

The talk was indeed "small" and woven into the mundane conversation of our daily lives. But it is one that I have to endure, relentlessly, over and over again. It is a question that reminds me that my body doesn't belong in certain spaces, for this question exposes the underlying and unspoken assumption that "you're not from here," from which the question "where are you from?" then logically follows. In other words, this question appears when there seems to be an uneasy disjuncture between the space, face, and race that the body-in-space exhibits. Hence, the question "where are you from?" brings to the surface both the relationships and tensions between places and racial categories and the ways in which bodies in motion and emotions expressed through these bodies become the link that glues the two categories of place and race together. Simultaneously, the question "where are you from?" also exposes the desire to attach meanings to the otherwise racially/spatially illegible bodies and to locate the body-in-space on some existing map of racial categories.

Beyond exposing the link between space and race, the question "where are you from?" also gets at a deeper and more theoretical question that feminist studies scholar Elspeth Probyn has asked, "What is it that drags upon us as we move through space? How are different spaces historically formulated as conducive to some subjectivities and not others?" (2003, 290). Questioning this stickiness between subjectivities and spaces is important because such an attachment is problematic: as sociologist Nadia Kim pointed out, for example, the space of Asia has been a signifier that sticks to Asian American bodies and as such, she argues, Asian Americans continue to experience racism because of their association with "Asia" (2008, 5).

I am interested in charting the ways in which space and its spatial tropes, articulated through political, geographical, and emotional discourses, become "imperative" signifiers for people's subjectivity particularly at moments of circulations and encounters across different geographical boundaries. This chapter therefore builds on, albeit departs from, studies that look at the importance of space in the formation of subjectivity (Tuan 1974/1990; Cosgrove 1984; Daniels 1993; Kinsman 1995, 301; Berg and Kearns 1996, 103; Kusno 2000, 211; Appadurai 2003, 342; Harvey 2009, 170) in that it locates such a concern within the specific discourse of emotions. I thus ask: how do circulations and representations of emotions about (transnational) spaces function to construct a specific racial, skin color, and gendered subjectivity in post-independence Indonesia?

I answer this question by closely reading beauty (mostly skin-whitening creams and cosmetics) advertisements published in women's magazines after independence was achieved. These magazines include the Dutch women's magazines *De Huisvrouw in Indonesie* (1949) and *De Huisvrouw* (1951, 1954–1956), and the Indonesian language women's magazines *Dunia Wanita* (1952, 1956–1957), *Ketjantikan* (1953), *Wanita* (1949–1953, 1956–1957), *Pantjawarna* (1948, 1957–1959), *Puspa Wanita* (1958, 1960), *Suara Perwari* (1951, 1953–1955, 1957–1958), *Warta* (1959–1960), and *Femina* (1975–1998). In reading these ads, I trace the discursive meanings of spatial tropes and the ways in which they are attached to certain emotions and the ways in which they then signify the meanings of specific "races" of women. This chapter thus rides the waves of gendered nationalism, cultural studies of emotion, racial formation, and gender studies in exploring and making theoretical sense of the relationships among space-based subjectivity formation, emotion, and the formation of the Indonesian nation.

If I previously discussed how Dutch colonialism shifted the meanings of light skin in the Indies' women's beauty discourse to mean predominantly white-skinned Caucasian women, and how the Japanese occupation reconfigured these meanings of light skin to now include Asian whiteness as the beauty ideal, here I question how Indonesians then constructed themselves in relation to whiteness after they gained their independence on August 17, 1945. By way of my analysis of beauty ads, I argue that although Indonesians resisted the idea of whiteness at first, after the end of the Cold War, they began to construct their own "Indonesian white" beauty ideal. Interesting to note here is that although in the early years of nation building there were fewer ads for skin-whitening products (not surprising given Soekarno's racial views), Europe was still attached to positive affects in these beauty ads. Nonetheless, the development of an Indonesian white beauty took place when there were more contacts with the West (the United States).

It is important here that we keep in mind the point made already in the prior chapters: that the "white" in Indonesian white beauty refers to skin color and not necessarily "race" as in the U.S. context. My using the word "white" actually exposes the limitation of language in discussing the issue of race and skin color in a transnational context. As Indonesian feminist scholar Aquarini Prabasmoro points out, in the Indonesian language, "she is white" means "she has light skin"; "she is black" means "she has dark skin" (2003, 34). The words black and white here do not signify race. Seemingly oxymoronic concepts such as "black Dutch" (used to refer to the Ambonese people of eastern Indonesia, during the colonial period) or *bule kulit hitam*, meaning black Caucasians (Caucasians with tanned skin or light-skinned African Americans) have at times appeared in daily conversation, indicating that skin color is named and understood differently in Indonesia.

I define Indonesian white beauty as a modern and postcolonial construction of an ideal of women's beauty that emerges out of both a long process of encounters with and resistance to Dutch colonialism, Japanese occupation, and American cultural imperialism and attempts to strategically represent and position Indonesian women within a global racial hierarchy. As such, Indonesian white beauty disrupts, challenges, but simultaneously reaffirms white as the superior and most desirable color across nations. This construction of white beauty that is signified by the geographical concept of "Indonesia" provides evidence for the ways in which spatial tropes play an important role in the affective process of subjectivity formation.

WHITENESS IN THE NEWLY
INDEPENDENT NATION (1945-1965)

Prior to gaining their independence, early Indonesian nationalists had envisioned the creation of an Indonesian nation that was not racialized. In the mid-1930s, for example, Indonesian nationalists attempted to formulate "a non-racial concept of an Indonesian nation," arguing that nation and state were not related to race and that race was not a satisfying category in itself because no race was a "pure" race (Suryadinata 1981, 159). This is not at all to suggest that Indonesians did not recognize "race." For example, an article appearing in the January 1921 edition of *Soenting Melajoe*, a West Sumatran magazine for women categorized five races on earth: Mongolians with their slanted eyes such as in Japan and China; Caucasians, such as Europeans and Arabs with a high nose; Africans, with black skin and curly hair; red-skinned Indians, the "true American children"; and Malays, including people from Madagascar, the Phillippines, and Taiwan with yellow and brown skin (14). Nonetheless, these nationalists' desire to formulate a non-racial concept of national identity may suggest that it was resistance to rather than the ignoring of the pervasiveness of race in late-colonial lives that stimulated this particular formulation of nationality. While during the colonial period, resistance seemed to engender either a refusal to be engaged with race or the construction of some other color as desirable, following Indonesia's independence, this resistance was articulated in more complex and oftentimes contradictory ways.

Indonesia's first president Soekarno (1945–1965) is characterized as predominantly anti-Western and genuinely concerned with the issues of race and nation (and only to a certain extent, gender). Soekarno even requested that Lothrop Stoddard's book *The Rising Tide of Color against White-World Supremacy*, published in 1920, be translated into Indonesian out of his concern that Indonesians needed to know more about race. In a chapter of the Indonesian version of Stoddard's book that was an addition to the original resentment against the Western white race was obvious. Soekarno was indeed open about his anti-Western views and nearing the end of his presidency in 1964 he even told Western countries to "go to hell with your aid" (Mackie and MacIntyre 1994, 36).

This may explain why, under Soekarno's presidency, there were fewer products advertised for whitening one's skin than during the colonial period or during the Soeharto era. One of the very few ads that advertised whitening or bleaching cream was an ad published in a 1955 Dutch women's magazine that was circulated in Indonesia, *De Huisvrouw*, although the caption itself was written in French (*incomparable pour blanchir et adoucir la peau*). Most other beauty ads simply used words such as "radiant" and "bright" (Indonesian, *bersinar terang* or *bercahaya terang*) to describe the desirable end result of these products. For example, an ad for Bi Yong Hoen powder that appeared in the magazine *Pantjawarna* in 1948 claimed to make one's face "sweet, smooth, young, and bright" (*manis, haluskan kulit, dan awet muda bercahaya terang*). Similarly, an ad published in *Pantjawarna* in 1958 for Djamu Galian Putri claimed that this traditional herbal beverage could make one's face "radiantly bright" (*bersinar terang*). Going a step further, an article published in *Warta* (1959) advised women to do a soft "bleaching" to "improve" their skin color, hinting at a white, but not too white, ideal skin color. Nonetheless, all of these examples suggest that although desire for whiteness is less frequently articulated in ads, bright/light skin was still affectively preferable even during the Soekarno era.

What happened in these ads were the conflation and the borrowing of meanings attached to "lightness" and "brightness" to signify the color of white. This conflation between lightness, brightness, and whiteness is interesting and has political and racial implications. In the Indonesian context, the metaphors of "light, dawn, and sun" have been used to represent "revival and regeneration" (Anderson 1990, 269). These metaphors were so popular that approximately a quarter of Indonesian newspapers from 1900–1925 used some reference to light in their titles, including sun, star, flame, or radiance (Anderson 1990, 243). Even the title of Indonesian early feminist Kartini's book, *Habis Gelap Terbitlah Terang* (*After Darkness, Light is Born*) uses this metaphor of brightness and darkness to mark a shift in Indonesian history from tradition to modernity (Anderson 1990, 243–244). Thus, the concept of bright (*terang*) has been used to highlight enlightenment, new consciousness, and a progression away from "darkness" (*gelap*), which has been framed as something that is undesirable.[1] In a sense, therefore, brightness, lightness, and whiteness were and still are metaphors important not only in beauty and racial discourses but also in narratives of modern Indonesian history because they figure as signifiers for the path to modernity. Moreover, particularly important to note for this chapter is that whiteness, brightness, and lightness are also spatial and temporal metaphors. That is, people imagine the space of darkness as scary and the space of lightness as good. The space of modernity therefore is an "enlightened" space.

The working of lightness, brightness, and whiteness to highlight progress in Indonesia is similar to and can be found in other cultures. For example, in Anglophone culture, lightness stands for knowledge (Mackie 1994, 130). In Japan, lightness is often used to mark political transformation and figured as "individual liberation" (Mackie 1994, 130–131, 133). Thus, whereas lightness represents freedom and class privilege, darkness represents its absence, confusion, threatening situations, and the working class. This relationship between class and lightness figured well, particularly in 1920s and 1930s Japan, by how the privileged class, a rich man and his mistress, for instance, were represented through shining objects (Mackie 1994, 133). Thus it is interesting to note that in Japan as in Indonesia, skin color marks one's class status, providing yet more evidence of the transnational construction and meanings of skin color and its signification to class standing.

Nonetheless, this refusal to use the word "white" and instead using other words to signify light skin color, mirrors the strategy used during the colonial period when, in resisting white as the dominant color, Indonesians used "yellow" to reaffirm the light-skinned beauty ideal. Indeed, history recorded that even during the colonial period there was already early resistance to white as the preferred skin color. In a serial story, "Nyai Ratna," published in *Medan Prijaji* in 1909, for example, Tirto Adhi Soerjo, an important Indonesian nationalist who later became the prototype of Pramoedya's *Buru* novels' character Minke, described the beautiful Nyai Ratna as "true, not white, but yellow" (Toer 1985, 301). In describing Nyai Ratna as "not white," the text posits white as the dominant skin color that it attempts to challenge. "Yellow" then became a "colored" space to resist this dominant color, a refusal of the text to accept beauty as defined by the colonizer. Yet, yellow was nonetheless another light skin color, which makes the text still complicit with the light-skinned beauty ideal. This resistance to the colonial ideal of beauty, which nonetheless reaffirmed an ideal light-skinned beauty, could also be found in periodicals such as *Bintang Hindia* (1928) whose images of "beautiful Javanese girls" (*Nona Jawa yang cantik manis*) were never images of dark-skinned women from eastern Indonesia.

Surprisingly, although Soekarno's policy was anti-Western and there were fewer products that claimed to "whiten"[2] one's skin, the images of women in magazines such as the Indonesian *Pantjawarna* and Dutch *De Huisvrouw* were still mostly European-descent Indo, if not Caucasian. This becomes all the more evident in this period because, unlike under colonialism when ads were composed of mostly text, with some sketch drawings, now more black and white photographic illustrations were used, making it easier to "see" who were considered truly beautiful and to whom positive affects were attached. For example, Lux still used Hollywood movie stars such as Joan Caulfield (1949), Jeanne Crain (1951), Ruth Roman (1956), and Belinda Lee (1957) to advertise their beauty soap. Ads for other beauty products, such as Vinolia talcum powder and Pond's cold cream, also used Caucasian women as models. Although Caucasian and Indo women continued to dominate the faces of beauty in Indonesia, in 1959 an Indonesian movie star, Dhiana, began advertising for Lux. This shift, I argue, was related to the nationalization of private corporations throughout 1957 and 1958 (Lindblad 1994, 212; Mackie 1994, 336). That is, after Indonesia's independence in 1945, the Dutch continued to play a significant role in Indonesia's economy. As economist Thee Kian Wie noted in his study, the Dutch occupied senior positions in the Indonesian public and financial sectors (1996, 316). As a response, the Soekarno government then nationalized some businesses: Java Bank, public utilities including gas and electricity companies, the airline, and railroads, were all nationalized in 1953. This nationalization continued until 1963 when all remaining British and American companies were nationalized. This thus put an end to foreign private enterprises in Indonesia that had been established since the colonial era.

The New Space of White Beauty

One can also detect the uneven development of Indonesian nationalism by considering the ways in which spatial tropes were used to signify a particular kind of beauty ideal. Atkinsons English Lavender Water and English Lavender Brilliantine, for example, consistently marked its ads with spatial tropes, specifically those of England, to highlight its superior quality and ability to bring happiness. In one of their ads, published in *Puspa Wanita* in 1958, the English caption that accompanies the black and white sketch drawing describes the "Song of Summer":

> Green leaves whispering, grey stones dozing . . . a limpid sky, the lovely breath of a thousand flowers . . . a dreamily happy mood punctuated with a brisk fragrance . . . Atkinsons English Lavender has it all.

In this ad, a "happy mood" is attached to the commodity Atkinsons English Lavender, with all of England's lovely summer contained in the bottle. In other words, its desirability is qualified by its association to England. Thus, the spatial "environment" of England, represented in this ad through its "limpid sky" and "the lovely breath of a thousand flowers," provides "the sensory stimuli, which as perceived images lend shape to our joys and ideals" (Tuan 1974/1990, 113).

Similarly, in an ad for the toothpaste Pepsodent published in *Puspa Wanita* in 1958, a Swiss woman is represented as smiling, showing off her beautifully white teeth. The caption that accompanies the ad reads, "This is the smile from Lucerne. . . . Whiter teeth in a week. Smiles of the girls from the beautiful Alps, Switzerland, are attractively sweet because of Pepsodent. Their teeth are shining white! This is also possible in Indonesia because Pepsodent is known the world over. . . . Special white teeth . . . in all countries." Here, the beautiful place of the Alps in Switzerland signifies the beautiful smile—a distinct smile "from Lucerne." In this ad, space becomes an important signifier for the people living in that place. Space functions as "a medium for reconnecting us with the material" (Kirby 1993, 175).

In other words, the concept of race is materialized, made "real" and "concretized," through the ways in which it is fixed in space (Pred 2000, 98–99). Historically, for example, processes of racialization have been expressed and regulated through space. As I've mentioned, in colonial Indonesia the "pass and quarter" system regulated and constructed race by naming which people could live and travel to which places. Such a control over space as an apparatus of racialization is called "spatial tactics": "the use of space as a strategy and/or technique of power and social control . . . the way space is used to obscure these relationships" (Low and Zuniga-Lawrence 2003, 30). In that sense, according to Allan Pred, writing about space and race in Sweden, "the social construction of race becomes one with the physical occupation of space" (2000, 98). Similarly, George Lipsitz writing of the American context notes, "the lived experience of race has a spatial dimension, and the lived experience of space has a racial dimension" (2007, 12). This organization of space based on race and the working of spatial tropes to signify race exemplify what sociologist Philip Cohen (1994) calls the "spatialization of race." In these ads, spatialization of race is evident by way of their employing spatial tropes (imbued with specific affective meanings) and using them to provide meanings for the race of the people living in those spaces, for example women in Switzerland are beautiful and desirable (and clean) because of their shining white teeth.

Attaching specific affective meanings to certain places inevitably creates problems. Framing Europe as the "source" of beauty in these ads necessarily produces and imposes social hierarchies among different countries and cities. In an ad, also for English Lavender, published in *Dunia Wanita* in 1956, the caption reads:

A new fragrance has come to this country . . . a fragrance so sweet, so smilingly young, that it could only have been born in the gardens of England. Soil, sun and tender care have nurtured that glorious flower called lavender, ever since the art of graceful living was practiced in the ancient manors of Britain. While Napoleon plotted the conquest of England, the firm of Atkinsons was becoming established. Here they learned how to capture this precious fragrance of English lavender and sent it out, to England, to Europe, to the Americas . . . to the dressing tables of leaders in the realm of charm and fashion. And now it comes to you! Atkinsons English Lavender Water and English Lavender Brilliantine can be obtained in every quality shop in Indonesia . . . at last!

This text highlights that although Indonesia is not the source of the beautiful product, it can now be a part of these great places because the product has arrived in Indonesia, "at last!" (A similar sentiment is expressed in an article published in *Puspa Wanita* [1958], stating that Paris is the number one city for fashion, whereas Hollywood was the second best [162], indicating a hierarchy for fashionable cities.) The English Lavender ad claims that its superior quality "could only have been born in the gardens of England," and nowhere else. This sense of England as the superior land is problematic, of course, because it hints at and is revealing of another hierarchy of power: among people living in these different places. To recall geographer Michael Brown's argument, "spatial metaphors and references can convey the relational sense of social relations (class, gender, sexuality, 'race,' etc.) and the identities that pole them" (2006, 319–320). Thus, such a reference to the "gardens of England" as simply the best possible place where such a desirable product could be produced carries with it traces of British (the people) imperial superiority, superior even compared to France's Napoleon.

Against a dominant narrative that positioned imported products as better than Indonesian products, however, there appeared also to be a counternarrative. An article in *Wanita* (1950) suggested that in the past women had not used imported cosmetics; to keep their skin smooth and "yellow" (*kuning langsep*), they had used what their grandmothers had made for them (253). Another article in the same magazine (*Wanita* 1950) made a similar suggestion for women who could not buy imported cosmetics: they should return to traditional homemade beauty recipes (232). Such a sentiment can also be seen in beauty ads such as that for the Indonesian-produced beauty powder Lily (*Wanita* 1950), that claimed that the quality of this product was as good as imported products while its price was more affordable.

Thus far I have demonstrated that space functions as a crucial signifier for the people occupying the space. But what do we make of this signifier–signified relationship between space and race? I would like to propose a concept that I call "emotionscape" to highlight the relationship between space and race that is imbued with emotions. In other words, I argue that the attachment between the concept of space and race is registered through the apparatus of emotions.

In developing the notion of emotionscape, I purposefully employ the suffix "-scape." First, "the term '-scape' implies there is a relationship between person and environment" (Houston quoted in Rodaway 1994, 64). Here, I think along the theoretical line of the landscape as "a way of experiencing and expressing feelings towards the external world, natural and man-made, an articulation of a human relationship with it" (Cosgrove 1984, 9). Emotionscape thus highlights the ways in which emotions "may be spatially ordered and place-related" (Porteus 1985, 369). The ads I discuss above, for example, show how feelings of happiness are attached to specific spaces such as England and Switzerland. Certain places may incite specific affective results.

Second, I use the suffix -scape to engage anthropologist Arjun Appadurai's (1996) notion of ideoscapes, financescapes, ethnoscapes, mediascapes, and technoscapes (global circulation of ideology, finance and capital, people, media, technology). In this sense, I offer emotionscape to help us think about the production of affective scripts—narratives of how we are supposed to feel—as an effect of global circulation of feelings, images, ideas, and people. Emotionscape thus emphasizes the ways in which emotions—not only ideology, finance, people, media, and technology—matter in processes of globalization. Emotionscape also functions as a repertoire of emotions from which people build their *imagined worlds* in this transnational age. Appadurai explains his use of the suffix -scape:

> These terms with the common suffix -*scape* also indicate that these are not objectively given relations that look the same from every angle of vision, but rather, that they are deeply perspectival constructs, inflected by the historical, linguistic, and political situatedness of different sorts of actors: nation-states, multinationals, diasporic communities, as well as subnational groupings and movements (whether religious, political, or economic), and even intimate face-to-face groups, such as villages, neighborhoods, and families. (1996, 33)

Thus, I am employing the suffix -scape in developing the concept emotionscape because, just as landscape is understood as "a perspectival construct," "a way of seeing," and a way of making meaning of, perceiving, and interpreting the visualized environment that is deeply influenced by political, historical, and other social contexts (Rodaway 1994, 129; Appadurai 1996, 33; Rose et al. 1997, 170), emotionscape is a mode of interpreting how emotions are visualized, interpreted, and made legible in spaces of representation, such as these ads. Historical and political shifts indeed affect the contour of emotionscape of white beauty in Indonesia, as I will explore in the next section.

THE NEW ORDER REGIME AND INDONESIAN WHITE BEAUTY (1966–1998)

Soekarno's successor, Soeharto, came to power in 1966 after a military coup a year earlier (backed by the U.S. Central Intelligence Agency) and remained president until 1998. That his coup was backed by a Western country signaled a significant change: the reentry of the West, particularly the United States, in Indonesian affairs. The "Guided Economy" or "Socialism à la Indonesia" policy, implemented under Soekarno, that no longer welcomed foreign private investments and tended to be more socialist, thus shifted in 1967 when Soeharto allowed, even encouraged, foreign direct investment in Indonesia (Mackie 1994, 336; Wie 1996, 328).

Unsurprisingly, Western ideologies soon began to dominate Indonesia's culture through various media. Foreign films, particularly from the United States, banned under Sukarno, reentered the market, threatening local production (Hatley 1994, 220). Women's magazines displayed glamorous global fashions surveying Western ideals of beauty. Changes in the economic sector were conspicuous. Foreign investment laws were shaped to accommodate, attract, and bring back foreign capital (Mackie and MacIntyre 1994, 35). Concessions were made between the Indonesian government and transnational companies. The 1970 oil boom gave way to "higher foreign exchange earnings and government revenues than Indonesia had ever experienced" (Mackie and MacIntyre 1994, 11–12).

Moreover, to create an image of an "investor-friendly" country and attract foreign investment, Soeharto repressed the labor movement at all cost. Repressing the labor movement was particularly important. Since the fall of international oil prices in the early 1980s, Indonesia has positioned itself as a producer of low wage, manufactured goods (Hadiz 2003, 96). The "class-based" labor movement, however, was not the only group to experience repression; people inside and outside academia were also prohibited from discussing or analyzing class (Farid 2005, 167–169, 189). Words like *buruh* (factory workers) were replaced by euphemisms such as *karyawan* or *pekerja* (office workers). This attempt to curb discussion of class was first couched within the discourse of anti-Communism at that time: it was the Indonesian Communist Party that employed class analysis in Indonesia (Farid 2005, 176). This partly explains why analysis of class in Indonesia has been limited.[3]

After Soeharto came to power, Indonesians living in big cities began to indulge in cosmopolitan consumerism in music, food, and fashion. Women's magazines that had become more profit-oriented after independence (Tomagola 1990, 64) now became even more so. What is interesting with the media environment around this time is that the Indonesian government issued a censorship policy, which was in effect in one way or another after 1960. Soeharto's policy was updated in a 1982 law requiring a license for publication[4] (Abidin 2005, 78). Although "censorship" was not named in this law, in practice a publication's license was simply revoked when it published articles that criticized the state, the president or his family; advocated what was deemed "communist" or "offensive" (albeit with unclear standards); or focused on ethnicity, religion, and race. Only in 1999 did Soeharto's successor establish freedom of the press by revoking the law requiring a government license (Abidin 2005, 23, 95).

Nonetheless, with the development of the printing industry, women's magazines grew significantly (Tomagola 1990, 68). This was the time when popular women's magazines such as *Femina* began publication. During its first year of publication in 1972, *Femina*, soon the most popular women's magazine in Indonesia, commonly represented Indonesian women alongside American women. Images even included women with "stereotypical" Indonesian facial features and a darker complexion. Such images appeared less often, year by year and had practically disappeared by the late 1990s.

As during the Soekarno era, under the Soeharto regime, spatial tropes continued to signify beauty ideals and the race that represents such space. During this time, Europe and the United States continued to be represented not only as the land of the beautiful, but also as the land from where authentic beauty comes. Ads with captions such as "Stendhal from Paris" (1978) and "Beauty Made in England" for Yardley (1979), "Swedish Formula Cosmetics" (1980), "Lancome Paris" (1980), and "Palmolive USA" (1984) were very common. Certainly, the places represented in these ads "invoke affective response according to practical and theoretical knowledges that have been derived from and coded by a host of sources" (Thrift 2004, 67–68). That is, in these ads, the marketability of the advertised products hinges on the audience's understanding of England and other European countries as affectively positive, represented as modern and technologically advanced, for instance. Here, the space is already affectively constructed prior to its being employed to signify the product.

In a Lux beauty soap ad published in *Femina* in 1978, the Indonesian movie star Widyawati was represented smiling as she stood in front of the Eiffel Tower wearing a "modern" outfit, including the French-style beret. The caption that accompanies the ad reads: "Every time I go to Paris, I always get the most advanced advice on the secret of beauty treatments. . . . I am very happy that the New Lux is now also available in Indonesia." Here, Paris is affectively evoked as a desirable and happy place for its beauty, modernity, and sophistication. Paris could even transform Widyawati's look, as she was represented in a more traditional way in other ads for the same beauty soap brand. Paris is also a place where she could get the most advanced beauty advice, which presumably she could not get in any cities in Indonesia. That Paris, and not any cities in Indonesia unless they carry Lux soap, can bring her happiness suggests that some places are perceived to be "more conducive to the generation of specific affective-emotional states than others" (Conradson and Latham 2007, 238). Paris is attached to what Conradson and Latham call the "affective possibilities" of a happy place.

Of course, these possibilities are just that, possibilities. No one can guarantee that everyone who visits Paris (or embodies Parisians by way of using Lux soap) will feel happy. These affective attachments are unpredictable (Sedgwick 2003, 62). No one can predict when or how a certain emotion can be attached successfully to a certain object. One may try, as in advertisements, to attach feelings of happiness to a beauty product, for instance, but no one can assure the audience that they will feel happy when they use the advertised product. This uncertainty surrounding the transfer of meanings and feelings reminds us of the discussion of *rasa* in chapter one: no one can truly guarantee that the audience will relish *rasa* when watching a performance. Nonetheless, although there is no guarantee that the audience will savor *rasa*, the production of *rasa* or emotion is not at all random (Thrift 2004, 68). The engineering of affects happens within these performances, or here, advertisements.

By representing Paris as a modern and happy place, an ad implicitly suggests that the emotionscape of Indonesia is an unhappy place, which could, however, become a happy place once New Lux, the object of desire, becomes available. Hence, Lux soap could only be perceived as a desirable object in Indonesia because of its European origin. Similarly, Indonesian whiteness that is constructed in this ad and embodied by Widyawati is articulated and legitimated through European whiteness. Indeed, even Widyawati herself, an Indo woman, embodies—literally—the partly European origin ideal. Here, Indonesian whiteness cannot claim its power affectively, given that the space of Indonesia is constructed as undesirable and unhappy. Even Indonesian whiteness must pass through Europe.

The emotionscape of white beauty in this ad presents white beauty as sophisticated and modern, represented by Paris and the Eiffel Tower, and attached to feelings of happiness. The place of France, or Paris, becomes a site where happiness resides:[5] "place or environment has become the carrier of emotionally charged events or perceived as symbol" (Tuan 1974/1990, 93). That is, as images of beauty and of places circulate transnationally, they carry with them the emotional meanings attached to these images. This is indeed one of the meanings of the concept of emotionscape that I develop, building on and adding to Appadurai's notion of five scapes. I argue that as emotions travel and circulate transnationally, they form a landscape—a repertoire and a repository—of dominant feelings about certain objects to which these emotions are attached. In this ad and in other beauty product ads, one of the dominant feelings of white feminine beauty is happiness. This ad suggests that to be beautifully white is to be happy, and to be happy, one must be beautifully white. However, according to this ad not any white beauty will do. This ad narrates that the white beauty that will bring happiness is European, or to be more specific, Parisian and white, signified by the spatial trope of the Eiffel Tower.

Another ad makes an even stronger claim of what kind of beauty would count as real beauty. The caption for a Yardley ad (1979), which shows a white Englishwoman smiling, says, "beauty made in England." In this ad, whiteness is embedded with positive affective quality, beauty, and boldly proclaims that this kind of beauty could only be made in England, not in Indonesia. Once again, the space of England is affectively constructed and constitutively represented as "good" prior to its meanings being embedded in the affective construction of the race of the model in the ad.

These beauty ads thus do the affective work of filling whiteness, England, or France, and whiteness in England or France with "positive," "feel-good" affective meanings. These ads also constitute the affective scripts that help structure our good feelings about places and people coming from these places (France, America, England, and Italy, for example). This consistent pattern of attaching certain emotions (i.e., happiness), to specific places (i.e., Europe), and objects (i.e., white beauty) provides evidence for the ways in which affect is not arbitrarily attached to things and therefore forms what I call the emotionscape of white beauty in transnational Indonesia. In all of these previously mentioned ads, race is figured through spatial tropes and space is therefore racialized. In other words, race is articulated through the affective meanings of spaces to which such race is tied. Race, I thus argue, is spatially expressed through affective registers *and* affectively expressed through spatial tropes.

Indonesian White Beauty and Skin-Whitening Products

That the space of Indonesia becomes a prominent and desirable signifier to provide meanings for "Indonesian white beauty" only comes later. Examining advertisements for skin-whitening products allows me to trace how and when this shift occurs. In the 1970s and early 1980s, ads for whitening products, including Tolino Pearl Cream (1975), Hinds Whitening Cream (1975), Kelly Pearl Cream (1976), Castella Soap (1977), Gizi Super Cream (1977), Vaeron Pearl Cream (1978), Fair Lady Cosmetic (1980), Juve Honey and Lemon Peeling Cream (1980), and Revlon Golden Pearl Skin Lightening Cream (1980), claimed only to diminish black spots rather than whiten the hue of the whole face or body. And some products, such as Tolino Pearl Cream, were also advertised for men. Yet, because the images in these ads were varied—an Asian man (Tolino Pearl Cream), a light-skinned Indian woman (Hinds Whitening Cream), a Caucasian woman (Vaeron Pearl Cream, Fair Lady Cosmetic, Revlon Golden Pearl Skin Lightening Cream), an Indo woman (Juve Honey and Lemon Peeling Cream, Castella Soap)—the "white" that these ads displayed was not yet Indonesian and the promised result not yet Indonesian white female beauty.

In the late 1980s, there began to be a shift in the language employed in these ads. More ads attempted to question the idea that European products were better by promoting Indonesian products as desirable. That is, beauty was more and more understood as "Indonesian." But to construct Indonesia as a desirable place, ads that marketed Indonesian products had to find a different route to attach positive affects to Indonesia. The most common signifiers employed in "Indonesian" beauty product ads were Indonesian natural settings, unmodernized spaces, and ethnic heritage homes. In other words, in these ads Indonesia is framed as the antithesis of the modern West. In some ads, Indonesia is even constructed as an "unreal," mythical place. In one Citra body lotion ad, published in *Femina* in 1987, seven women are bathing in the river. In the backdrop, a man is stealing the women's clothing. This scene evokes the ancient Javanese folktale of Jaka Tingkir and the celebrated beauty of the seven nymphs.

However, a careful reading of the ad's background reveals the legacy of colonialism. First, the image resembles colonial images that represent what historian Rudolf Mrázek calls the "beautiful Indies" that must not cast a shadow of troubles (1999, 40). To be perceived as the beautiful Indies, Mrázek argues, "a picture must contain no suggestion of waving time, no trembling of the air, no hidden energies, nothing hinted at in the shadows. The trees, houses, fields, mountains, and the people had to be distinctively outlined. The perspective should swell forward, and everything should offer itself to be seen" (1999, 40). The Citra ad exudes precisely this "beautiful Indies" energy, as can be seen from the ways the ad captures the perfect, idyllic state of the river and the women who leisurely bathe in such a sensuous body of water. Framed with(in) a colonial gaze, this ad, although it is not legitimated by the presence of a European white woman's body nor European spatial tropes, nonetheless relies on the European colonial gaze to justify the desirability of such a space.

Second, this imagined, mythical Indonesian space is represented as an affectively desirable place: unpolluted, untouched, and premodern. Indeed, the Indonesian village is often described as a site of good feelings and often romanticized through the notion "back to nature" (Malik 1997, 214). It also provides a sense of "authenticity" (Kusno 2000, 152). On the contrary, the city is often represented as a site of anxiety, tension, and alienation; Indonesian poets often attach negative feelings to cities (Malna 2000, 384). Evidently, in order to construct a positive feeling about Indonesia, the space signified as Indonesia had to be represented by a river, not a modern Indonesian city. In other words, European countries are evoked as desirable places precisely because of their modernity, but Indonesia can only be represented as desirable through its lack of modernity.[6]

By the 1990s, whitening product advertisements took on an even more specific discourse of female beauty: it was no longer Indonesians in general, but rather women only who were represented and invited to use whitening creams. Men were no longer considered a target market.[7] If men appeared at all in these ads, they functioned simply to admire the beauty of these now-whitened women. Indonesian white beauty had become a specifically gendered concept. Although whitening ads still incorporated claims that their product could prevent sun damage, they became more and more about women's self-improvement and achievement. For example, an ad for Pond's Fair and Lovely insinuated that by using this product one can, as the ad's title suggests, "prepare [herself] in the best possible manner to pursue [her] career."

I relate this change of language in ads to world politics, particularly the end of the Cold War in 1989. The supposed triumph of American capitalism contributed to two developments that occurred in Indonesia at this time: (1) the dissemination of an ideology of "rugged individualism" through and because of (2) the emergence of private television stations and television advertising. Indonesia's first private television station, RCTI (*Rajawali Citra Televisi Indonesia*), was founded in 1989 (by a group that included one of Soeharto's sons, Bambang Triatmojo). It first aired only regionally but then, in 1990, nationally. Another private television station, SCTV (*Surya Citra Televisi*) (whose owners included one of Soeharto's daughters), began broadcasting in several cities in East Java in 1990 and then nationally in 1993. Other private television stations started up at the turn of the twenty-first century.

As in Japan after the 1950s, when many families began to own private television sets and could watch stories about white middle-class Americans, "images of Whites on screen [became] 'natural'" (Creighton 1997, 216–217). In Indonesia after the Cold War whiteness was also naturalized and became the "norm" on television. The very popular U.S. films and TV series that traveled to Indonesia were usually, with the exception of "The Cosby Show" (*Keluarga Pak Huxtable*), about middle-class white families. These shows and their ads oftentimes narrated stories about love and families and reinforced the idea that the individual was responsible for her own happiness, with "happiness" usually equated with looking good and being loved. Hence, what these shows also circulated was the ethic of rugged individualism. Moreover, with the language of self-transformation that presumes that beauty is a personal/individual responsibility, ugliness then becomes the fault of the individual. Compare this to the ideology of the Japanese occupation when beauty was represented as "women's duty" for the nation and her husband; after the Cold War, beauty becomes a responsibility to help women achieve some self-interest such as a career or love.

Certainly, even prior to 1989, Indonesia's public TV station already aired American films and TV series, but there were fewer then compared to what new private TV stations made possible. And because having only one TV station limited the development of Indonesian films and TV series prior to 1989, these new spaces were first filled with mostly American and to a lesser extent Indian films and Spanish telenovelas. All of these, including Indian films with their light-skinned movie stars, as well as (whitening) advertisements on television, served to reinforce white/light skin as the most desirable color.

However, during this period when the world seemed to become more open and accessible through the medium of television, the need to define oneself against others became more important. That is, while whiteness became the norm, there was a need to define an *Indonesian* version of whiteness. Hence, constructing Indonesian white beauty was a way to negotiate the representation of the face of the nation in a transnational age. For these corporations, the way to distinguish "Indonesian women" from "other" women was to convince targeted women that their products are for them, the Indonesian women. Whitening ads, for example, were specific in invoking the Indonesianness of white skin color. Ads such as Sari Ayu-Martha Tilaar's Pelembab Putri Matari (1995), Mustika Ratu's Masker Bengkoang (1996–), and Citra White Lotion (1996–) used signifiers such as flowers, traditional clothing, or a tropical setting to highlight their (traditional) Indonesianness. Signifying their products as Indonesian was particularly important for Citra White Lotion, which in 1989 still used the word "yellow" (*kuning langsat*) but then changed and used the word "white" (*putih*) instead to name the desirable skin color in advertising another one of their beauty products, Citra Beauty Lotion. This Indonesian (nation as) signifier was an attempt to assure its target market that the company's move to produce whitening products was still within the boundaries of creating an "Indonesian white beauty" for Indonesian women.

It is worthy to note here that in these ads, the spaces that were signified to stand for the national identity had to be "traditionalized" first. An ad for Sariayu Koleksi Samudra Pasai and Koleksi Gayo, published in *Femina* in 1996 exemplifies this point clearly. It starts off with four paragraphs describing the magnificence of the spaces that are used as the labels of the cosmetics:

> From Samudra Pasai to the hills of Gayo. . . . the history of Aceh records Peurlak as the oldest Islamic kingdom in Indonesia, which was then followed by the golden years of Samudra Pasai.
>
> Its fame and beauty made Aceh the intersection of different cultures. In 1292 Marco Polo in his journey to find spices made a sojourn in Aceh for months. During this time, Aceh's black pepper was the treasure that was sought after by the world.
>
> Aceh is a cultural rainbow that would not vanish. Its carvings decorate its parks. Its knitting decorate the clothing. Gold and jewels decorate various jewelries as beautiful melodies accompany its dances.

Aceh's nature is like a landscape painting that is rich with color and nuances. The grandeur of Mount Seulawah. The white sands. Hilly Gayo's coffee plantation and fruits. Laut Tawar Lake circled with pine tree forest and surrounded by different flowerbeds.

Here, the evocation of the past, i.e., the grandeur of "Samudra Pasai" as an Islamic kingdom in the thirteenth century, functions to evoke nostalgia for an idyllic place. As Tuan pointed out, "patriotic rhetoric has always stressed the roots of a people" (1974/1990, 99). Hence, these paragraphs function to emphasize such roots and to signify the space of Aceh with positive affects such as love and admiration. Along with the background images of the "traditional" houses of the Acehnese and women dressed in traditional Acehnese clothing, they are part of the "traditionalizing" process. This process, according to geographer Brenda Yeoh, is an element of the postcolonial nation's strategy: "the selective retrieval and appropriation of indigenous and colonial cultures to produce appropriate forms to represent the postcolonial present" (2003, 371). In other words, by way of its being represented through traditional clothing and housing images in this ad, Aceh *becomes* a "traditional" space. Aceh is not a place of heritage prior to or outside of its representation.

The beginning four paragraphs are directly followed by two paragraphs that boast of Acehnese women and therefore join the signifiers of the place and people together:

Acehnese women dazzle with their own beauty. Ratu Nahrasiyah from Samudra Pasai ruled with wisdom. Laksamana Keumalahayati led the attack and defeated Cornelius de Houtman's army. Cut Nyak Dien never gave up in her struggles against colonialism.

The behavior of Acehnese women should be the role models for contemporary Indonesian women. They stand equal to men in their dedication to the Motherland. Nonetheless, they understand their place as mothers in the family. It is an attitude that women all over the world give important attention to. It is a spirit that becomes the foundation for the creation of the color trend for contemporary Indonesian women.

Hence, in these ads, the place of Aceh and the women living in magnificent Aceh stand for each other and the meanings of one are transferred to the other. The space becomes an extension of or a credible signifier for the Acehnese women's personality, which then becomes the signifier for the advertised product. It is indeed through these descriptions of the space of Aceh and its women that the emotionscape of Indonesian white beauty is produced and circulated.

Beyond constructing the Indonesian (space-based) nation as a signifier for the product, there is another way in which these ads assured Indonesian women that these products were for them: by using Indonesian women, mostly Indo women, instead of Caucasian women who previously had been used to advertise various beauty products including whitening creams, in their ads. (This phenomenon of using Indonesian women to model for skin-whitening ads is specific to this period. As can be seen in the next chapter, the models for skin-whitening ads in post-reform twenty-first-century Indonesia were women coming from different racial and national backgrounds.) There are several reasons why Indo women became the perfect embodiment of Indonesian white beauty during this period. First, as political scientist William R. Liddle (1996) argues, Indonesian national culture is one that values both native and modernized Western culture. Hence it is Indo women—both native and Western—who become the perfect embodiment of beauty. Second, as Prabasmoro, who has examined how Indo women and their bodies have come to represent an ideal beauty, emphasizes, the Indo woman "could only be white in a non-white culture." Prabasmoro calls Indonesia a "non-white" (*bukan putih*) society. She explicitly says that she is willing to take the risk of claiming Indonesia as a "non-white" culture by arguing that "because Indonesians don't think of themselves as white or black as is understood within the dichotomy of white/black races, . . . it is more accurate to say that Indonesian culture and bodies are not white and not black rather than to affirm that it is part of either one" (Prabasmoro 2003, 35). However, her argument overlooks the fact that people of "white" and "black" races also are Indonesian citizens and that Indonesians do, particularly in regard to skin color, desire whiteness, albeit an Indonesian whiteness. She writes,

> As is implied by universality, white is a color that consists of other colors. White is the sum of all colors; it is a non-color/yet all colors. In the case of Indo celebrities in soap ads, I find that white skin color is emphasized in such a way that their whiteness hides their other colors (non-white color) while simultaneously reaffirming their partial whiteness. . . . Hence, in the local context, the representation of this non-white body is accepted to be white enough, although it is not white enough to be white in the global context. (Prabasmoro 2003, 91)

That Indo women are being perceived as not embodying white skin color in a global context is signified by their race and nation—Asian and Indonesian. Simultaneously, their being accepted as representing an Indonesian white beauty ideal in the local context is driven by the fact that they are indeed Indonesians, by race and nationality. That is, here, it is once again the "space-based" identity that gives meaning to their skin color.

To further build on Prabasmoro's argument, however, I would point out that it is precisely the ability of these Indo women to be simultaneously white and non-white that functions as a subversive power. Whiteness, as Alastair Bonnett points out, can be "redeployed" to be "subversive" (2002, 98). The presence of these white-but-not-white female bodies on television shows, in magazines, and in ads challenges and interrupts the Caucasian American white beauty ideal narratives also present in these same media. Particularly because "white people are who white people say are white . . . has a profoundly controlling effect" (Dyer 1997, 48), to claim that Indonesian women are white and yet their whiteness is different from or even better than Caucasians is powerful for it rejects the control of whites to claim that they are the only whites there are.

But if the process of constructing a beauty ideal is used not only for the commercial purpose of selling beauty products but also for the purpose of constructing a gender-based national identity, it involves not only a question of whose faces have been included but also who is and what does this tell us about Indonesian national identity. It is here that the question of the invisibility of dark-skinned women particularly from eastern Indonesia arises.

Why are women from eastern Indonesia or Indonesian women of African descent omitted from this beauty ideal that stems from the larger national narrative? There are a couple of possible explanations. First, women from eastern Indonesia and/or of African descent are rarely incorporated into Indonesian history. Even one of the most comprehensive books on Indonesian history, historian Jean Gelman Taylor's *Indonesia: Peoples and Histories*, overlooks the presence of people of African origin in Indonesian history. This omission exists despite the fact that African descendants in the Indonesian archipelago are confirmed by twelfth-century *prasasti* (stone relics) that recorded the existence of zangi people possibly from East Africa (Derideaux 2006). Or, if the presence of people (not necessarily women) of African descent appears at all, such as in the book *Pasang Surut*, they are represented as "primitives" (*Pasang Surut* 276–277). It is particularly striking that European men living in colonial Batavia rarely married African women, although they were "abundantly present at that time," but did marry dark-skinned Portuguese-speaking women of Indian origin (Blussé 1986, 156; Raben 1996, 283–284). This suggests that skin color is not the determining factor in marriage. Rather, the ways in which the meanings of race, as it is dissociated from skin color, signify the cultural understandings of a particular skin color influence the marriageability factor of women with dark skin color.

Second, within the narrative of nationalism, a dominant beauty ideal does the work of serving the interests of its ruling elites. Southeast Asian studies scholar Ingrid Wessel points out that nationalism works to "stabil[ize] and justi[fy] the ruling elite" (1994, 39). The ruling elites have an interest in maintaining the omission and controlling the representations of women (and men) from eastern Indonesia and/or African descent in Indonesia. This seems to be what Ani Sekarningsih (2000) in her novel *Namaku Teweraut* attempts to address: how Javanese elites have benefited financially from representing eastern Indonesia (in her novel, people from *Asmat*) as "primitive." Here, the postcolonial nation's dialogue with its own "colonial past has resulted . . . in the reproduction of a form of colonialism itself" (Kusno 2000, 212). That is, as Asian studies scholar Abidin Kusno argues, the new nation, in reimagining its postcolonial identity, seems to become a colonizer itself, albeit a different version of it. Narratives of nationalism function as the new master's apparatus to "colonize" its own postcolonial nation. This exclusion of dark-skinned eastern Indonesian women thus exposes the limit of "national imagination" in imagining a particular kind of whiteness as an ideal representation of Indonesia. Such an imagining of specific Indonesian white beauty, as I will discuss in chapter five, also hides and marginalizes Chinese-Indonesian women whose skin color might be lighter than other women in Indonesia yet are also excluded from such an imagining.

This chapter thus traces the troubling ways in which the postcolonial nation came to be formed (and transformed) out of the constantly shifting representations of women's beauty as they are framed within the discourse of gender, whiteness, and the foreign yet "superior" lands of Europe and America. Moreover, I have also shown both continuity and discontinuity of power and representation in the different phases of political regimes in postcolonial Indonesia. As such, I have exposed the difficulty (not the stability) of portraying whiteness in different periods in Indonesia.

CONCLUSION

In conclusion, I return to my main point: the ways in which narratives of gendered and racialized nation have been articulated through space. That is, around the time when the postcolonial nation was in the process of reimagining and building itself, "space" became central to the formation of identity. Space takes on an important role during this particular time because during the postcolonial period, unlike during the precolonial and colonial periods, claiming one's identity was also about claiming one's national space. Indeed, as anthropologist Akhil Gupta argues, "nation" is "the hegemonic form of organizing space," national identity is "an expression of identity that reflects one's spatial commitment," and nationalism is "a new kind of spatial and mythopoetic meta-narrative" (2003, 321, 329, 332). Similarly, Appadurai articulates such a point: "discourses of nationalism remain the vessels for the ideology of territorial nationalism" (2003, 342). Speaking specifically about the Indonesian context, Asian studies scholars Michael Hitchcock and Victor King point out how the Indonesian nation is constructed through one's awareness of its spatial continuity and presence:

> A vital element in the formation of national consciousness was the development of an awareness of the spatial continuity of Indonesian territory. A nation's identity is often closely linked to definitions of space, a defined territory forming an imaginary community that exists in a given location. It comprises an information network of signs and symbols, in which the borders correspond with an exclusive body of identity markers. (1997, 4)

All of these points highlight the ways in which space and place function as a mode of categorizing and thinking about different identities such as national identities and, in this chapter, gendered racial identities.

In essence, this chapter highlights the centrality of affective production about certain "spaces of representation" in constructing race and gender affectively. It provides a critical reading of beauty ads published in women's magazines to reveal how the deployment of spatial tropes in these ads is implicit in and relies on the production of *rasa* about these places, the people who inhabit these places, and therefore the racial categories that are signified by them. In these ads, one of the ways in which race is constructed affectively is through how we *feel* about these spaces that are then deployed as signifiers that provide meanings for people living in these spaces and the racial categories that are embedded in these meanings. Spatial tropes thus materialize and visualize such racial categories and the beauty that certain races of people embody. This means that these spatial tropes "are used in ways that link psychological states of mind and being with physical location, situation and movement" (Brown 2006, 321). In other words, space functions as a signifier for the production of specific feelings: "affective states come to be associated with particular places" (Conradson and Latham 2007, 238).

Highlighting the importance of spatial tropes that provide meanings for race and skin color, I have provided evidence for how the construction of the gendered and racialized category of identity, specifically Indonesian white beauty, relies on the manipulation of feelings about certain places. Space thus functions as a locus of affective production and subjectivity formation. More-over, by theorizing the construction of Indonesian white beauty, I argue that whiteness need not be Caucasian race only—note that Caucasian itself also derives from the *place* of Mount Caucasus—but rather can and has referred specifically to skin color.

4 | *Cosmopolitan* Whiteness

The Effects and Affects of Skin-Whitening Advertisements in a Transnational Women's Magazine

In the June 2006 edition of the Indonesian version of the magazine *Cosmopolitan* (hereafter referred to as *Cosmo*), Estée Lauder's "Cyber White" ad appeared on the inside front-cover spread of the magazine. In the following issue of the Indonesian *Cosmo* (July 2006) Kosé's Sekkisei whitening ad with the slogan "Skin of Innocence" appeared as the front-cover gatefold. Interestingly, in the late 1980s and 1990s when the preference for light skin color was visually represented by "Indonesian white" women, neither of these transnational ads employed Indonesian models: a Caucasian woman models the "Cyber White" ad and a Japanese woman models the Sekkisei ad. These skin-whitening ads, modeled by women of different racial backgrounds and facial features, raise the question: what kind of whiteness is being marketed in transnational women's magazines?

Thus, in this chapter, I look at post-Soeharto (post-1998) Indonesia, specifically 2006–2008, to answer this question and demonstrate a further shift in meaning of whiteness in contemporary Indonesia. That is, although the preference for light-skinned women precedes European colonialism and continued after Indonesia's independence, the meanings of light skin color throughout these different historical periods varied significantly. In our contemporary moment, light-skinned women are resignified: no longer just "Caucasian white" as in the Dutch colonial period, nor "Japanese white" as during the occupation, nor "Indonesian white" as in the decades following independence, but something more complicated that I call "*cosmopolitan* whiteness." (I use "cosmopolitan" here both in refererence to the magazine's title and for its larger meaning.)

Existing studies on the skin-whitening phenomenon in a variety of countries fall short of answering this question because they operate under the assumption that whiteness is an ethnic or racially based category, however marked it may be by biological, social, and visual signifiers (Burke 1996; Peiss 1998; Kawashima 2002; R. Hall 2005; M. Hunter 2005; Rondilla and Spickard 2007; Pierre 2008; Glenn 2009; Parameswaran and Cardoza 2009). For example, when cultural studies scholar Radhika Parameswaran and journalist Kavitha Cardoza point out that whitening advertisements in contemporary Indian media do not necessarily reveal women's desire to be racially white, they are equating "white" with racially Caucasian people (2009). Similarly, when historian Timothy Burke notes that women's consumption of skin whiteners in modern Zimbabwe was considered a sign of (re)colonization and "selling-out" to the white regime, he also positioned "white" as a racial category (1996). Indeed, the term "white-privileging subject position" that Asian studies scholar Terry Kawashima coined in her analysis of contemporary anime, skin-whitening ads and hair-coloring pratices in Japan also rest on the same assumed white racial category: Caucasian (2002).

Other important studies on the racial politics of beauty that challenge body-altering practices as merely revealing people's desires for the white beauty norm nonetheless refer to Caucasian whiteness as a frame for referencing "whiteness." Kathleen Zane, although providing us with a different way of reading Asian women's eyelid surgeries that goes beyond Asian women's desire to "imitate a Caucasian appearance" (1998, 355), still attaches the category of Caucasian whiteness to the meaning of a white beauty norm. Race and cultural studies scholar Kobena Mercer has demonstrated the complex "inter-culturation" of so-called "artificial" and "natural" techniques of hairstyling among black people (as well as among people in "white subcultures") and asks "whom in this postmodern mêlée of semiotic appropriation and counter-creolization, is imitating whom?" (1987, 52). Yet he also refers to Caucasian whiteness when he highlights this complexity of whiteness as an embodied racial category. Thus, although critical scholarship on the racial politics of beauty convincingly debunks the myth of racially authentic bodies and points to the unstable quality of "looking white," these studies nonetheless still subscribe to the very notion of Caucasian whiteness as the point of theoretical reference in challenging such whiteness.

This chapter breaks away from these theoretical trajectories by arguing that desire for "whiteness" is *not* the same as desire for "Caucasian whiteness." By examining skin-whitening advertisements in the Indonesian *Cosmo* published during the months of June, July, and August, 2006–2008,[1] I argue that in contemporary Indonesia, there has been a shift from Indonesian white beauty toward what I am calling "cosmopolitan whiteness." By cosmopolitan whiteness, I refer to a whiteness that is represented to embody the "affective" and virtual quality of cosmopolitanism: transnational mobility. Here affect is understood as preceding emotions, yet also involving "sociality or social productivity" (Wissinger 2007, 232). I position these ads as a socially productive site where affective qualities about white-skinned women are produced, represented, and circulated.

I propose the notion of cosmopolitan whiteness as a mode for rethinking whiteness beyond racial and ethnic categories and for thinking about race, skin color, and gender as "affectively" constructed. To think about whiteness beyond a racial or ethnic category is not to argue that race and racialization are irrelevant in thinking about whiteness, of course. Rather, I argue that whiteness is *also* affectively constructed as cosmopolitan and that race and racialization operate in concert with cosmopolitanism in these whitening advertisements.

Redefining whiteness as cosmopolitan whiteness allows me to reveal yet another aspect of cosmopolitanism *and* whiteness that is not often discussed: its virtuality. Virtuality here is understood as occupying the space between the real and the unreal—the virtual. This notion of virtuality is important in understanding cosmopolitan whiteness because virtuality highlights the lack of "traditional physical substance" (Laurel 1993, 8). I argue that cosmopolitan whiteness is a signifier without a racialized, signified body. Cosmopolitan whiteness can and has been modeled by women from Japan to South Korea to the United States. There is no one race or ethnic group in particular that can occupy an authentic cosmopolitan white location because there has never been a "real" whiteness to begin with: whiteness is a virtual quality, neither real nor unreal.

This chapter anchors its analysis of skin-whitening advertisements in affect theories and cultural studies of emotion; in doing so, it aims to advance our understanding of the ways in which race, gender, and skin color are not only socially and visually constructed but also affectively, virtually, and transnationally constructed. As such, it operates at the intersection of affect theories and cultural studies of emotions and theories of gendered racialization, transnationalization, and cyberculture studies and pays careful attention to the affective structures through which gender and race are constructed. Racialization processes rely on how people feel about others: "feeling" is where the structural and the individual collide.

My argument is drawn from a critical reading of advertisements for skin-whitening products published in the Indonesian version of the U.S. women's magazine *Cosmopolitan* and to a limited extent, advertisements of tanning products in the U.S. *Cosmo*. I chose the Indonesian and American *Cosmo* because it allows me to trace circulations of popular culture from the United States to Indonesia. I do so by examining the U.S. edition of *Cosmo* and by charting which images and articles "travel" from the United States to reappear in the Indonesian version of *Cosmo*. Simultaneously, because articles that contextualize these ads are the prerogative, in the Indonesian version, of an Indonesian editor, I also make visible the voices and agencies of Indonesians in circulating images and narratives pertinent to issues of skin color, gender, race, and sexuality in a transnational context.

In the following pages, I provide a context that addresses the politics of the transnational circulation of *Cosmo* from the United States to Indonesia. Such a context will help demonstrate how "a racially saturated field of visibility" (Butler 1993, 15) has limited the readings of skin-whitening ads as merely reflecting desires for Caucasian whiteness. This contextual grounding leads us directly into the analysis of these whitening ads, focusing on both the construction of cosmopolitan whiteness and on the ads as a site for the production of a cosmopolitan whiteness as something that is good and desirable. I do the latter by focusing on one exemplary ad, Estée Lauder's "Cyber White," to provide evidence for my argument that the construction of cosmopolitan whiteness contributes to the production of "positive" affects toward white-skinned women, that virtuality is an important aspect of cosmopolitan whiteness, and that the production of these "good" affects relies on the ads' "facialization" process. Finally, I will end this discussion on how cosmopolitan whiteness is reaffirmed even in tanning ads that market the idea of darker color as desirably beautiful.

TRANSNATIONAL CONTACTS AND *COSMO* CONTEXTS: THE COSMO POLITICS OF TRANSNATIONAL CIRCULATION FROM THE UNITED STATES TO INDONESIA

U.S. popular culture, from its films and magazines to its consumer products, has become one of the most powerful "nodes" shaping the terrain of contemporary Indonesian pop culture (Appadurai 1996). Comparing ads for similar products in a U.S. magazine and its Indonesian version also allows me to shift my analysis from Dutch and Japanese influences to the United States. Of course, Japanese popular culture still penetrates contemporary Indonesian culture along with popular American culture. Of further significance to my analysis is that the United States, as home to people from various nations and racial backgrounds, has different histories of race, gender, skin color, and sexuality from Indonesia's. This makes objects coming from the United States interesting sites of analysis for they allow us to investigate the ways in which politics of gender, race, skin color, and sexuality, which underpin the very production of the U.S. *Cosmo*, travel to and help reconfigure the politics represented in the Indonesian *Cosmo*.

Moreover, it is important to remember that the United States has played a significant role in Indonesian politics, particularly after Indonesia's formation as a nation-state in 1945. However, the political relations between these two countries, especially in the years immediately following Indonesia's independence, can be described as precarious at best. Indonesia certainly had every reason to distance itself from the United States, particularly because the United States provided weapons, trucks, planes, and financial support to the Dutch to recolonize Indonesia after World War II (Kahin and Kahin 1995, 30). And when the Dutch failed to reestablish its power in Indonesia, the United States, whose foreign policy at that time was fixated on eradicating Communism, attempted to undermine Soekarno's communist-leaning government. Hence, in the late 1950s the Eisenhower administration launched a covert effort to support various Indonesian separatist movements. Eisenhower's secretary of state, John Foster Dulles, even expressed that in order for the United States to eliminate Communism in Indonesia, it was in the United States' best interest to have Indonesia "disintegrated" rather than "united." However, following the "Allen Pope" incident,[2] the United States shifted its policy to support a compromise between the central government and "rebel" groups—at least until another strategy to eliminate Communism in Indonesia was devised (Kahin and Kahin 1995, 75, 203–204).

In 1965, the U.S. Central Intelligence Agency finally succeeded in ending the communist influence in Indonesia. The United States supported a pro-Western, pro-U.S. military general, Soeharto, in a coup that toppled Soekarno (La Botz 2001, 41). Soeharto then cooled Indonesia's relations with communist countries and banned the Indonesian Communist Party. Soeharto remained Indonesia's president for thirty-two years: his decision to voluntarily step down in 1998 following large-scale protests and the collapse of the economy was influenced in part because he lost the U.S. government's support. Since 1998, Indonesia has had four presidents and has been undergoing a democratization process.

Particularly since 1998, there has been a major boom in Indonesian adaptations of American magazines such as *Cosmo*, *Good Housekeeping*, and *Esquire*. Hence, although my focus is on examining skin-whitening ads in the Indonesian *Cosmo*, in this section, I will also look at the U.S. *Cosmo* during the same months (June–August of 2006–2008) to chart the circulation of beauty, racial, and gender discourses through this transnational magazine. Moreover, examining the United States as a site where whiteness is articulated as "desirable," my analysis makes visible how transnational circulations of whiteness from the United States to Indonesia depend on the ways in which whiteness is capable of maintaining its currency globally (hence the notion of cosmopolitan whiteness).

The magazine I examine here, *Cosmopolitan*, is one of the most popular transnational women's magazines in Indonesia. It originated in the United States in 1886 as a literary/fiction magazine. It underwent a significant transformation in 1965 when its new editor, Helen Gurley Brown, the well-known author of *Sex and the Single Girl*, took a daring step by shifting the magazine's focus to women's sexuality *and*, as well as *in*, the workplace (McMachon 1990; Spooner 2001). With the slogan, "fun . . . fearless . . . female," U.S. *Cosmo*'s strategy of marketing to and advocating for sexually independent women saved it from almost certain bankruptcy. Prior to 1965, sexuality was rarely discussed in U.S. women's magazines, which were focused more on women's place in the home (Nelson and Paek 2005). In Indonesia as well, when *Cosmo* (originally called *Kosmopolitan Higina*) first began publication in September 1997, promoting sexually assertive women (albeit in a much subtler way compared to the 2006–2008 editions that I analyzed) meant breaking new ground. Although some Muslim groups in Indonesia sent letters to the editor protesting that the magazine was "helping Indonesian women love sex too much" (Carr 2002), nonetheless, the strategy of putting forth women's independence through sexuality was what made *Cosmo* one of the most successful magazines in the world. It has fifty-eight international editions, is published in thirty-four languages, and is circulated in over one hundred countries. *Cosmo* is indeed the most popular transnational women's magazine in Indonesia, with a circulation of 139,000. In the Indonesian context, marketing specialist Hermawan Kartajaya applauded its marketing strategy, arguing that *Cosmo*, by carefully formulating and consistently encouraging women to adopt a "cosmopolitan woman" identity, provided a space for Indonesian women to reject society's masculine domination (2004).

From the eighteen issues of the Indonesian and U.S. *Cosmo* that I analyzed, I found that most articles and images in the two versions were different, although they seemed to be similarly structured and drew from similar sources. This is so because *Cosmo* is a transnational magazine with its own confidential "50-page manual, which dictates criteria in selection of cover models and editorial focus" (Nelson and Paek 2005, 372). For example, when both versions featured American celebrity/actress Brittany Murphy on their cover (July 2006 of American *Cosmo* and August 2006 of Indonesian *Cosmo*), she was photographed wearing different dresses. The Indonesian version shows her in a sexy, tight-fitting, red dress. The American version represents her in a colorful, floral-print tropical dress. Hence, although at first glance the two covers seem the same with the same celebrity and even feature articles on the same topics, the Indonesian *Cosmo* is not simply a direct translation of the U.S. *Cosmo*. Names are changed from American to Indonesian, and local examples or commentary by local experts are added in the Indonesian version. Based on research by media studies scholars David Machin and Joanna Thornborrow (2003), Michelle Nelson and Hye-Jin Paek (2005), and Jui-Shan Chang (2004) that examined *Cosmo* in several countries around the globe, this is not unique to the Indonesian case. From her work on Taiwan, for example, Chang concludes that the production of *Cosmo* is both centralized and localized: the various editions can borrow materials from the "central bank"—that is the New York headquarters—or from "sister" issues in other countries, as well as producing their own articles. Consequently, each issue of *Cosmopolitan* . . . contains a unique blend of global and local cultural ingredients on topics concerning modern womanhood. (2004, 363)

As such, the magazine not only uses the word "cosmopolitan" as a label to address its reader, the "cosmo" woman, it also embodies the very notion of cosmopolitanism by producing its magazines transnationally. It is these cosmopolitan meanings, deployed in various ways by *Cosmo*, in addition to the transnational formation of a racialized beauty ideal, that provide me with the context within which I read whitening ads published in the Indonesian *Cosmo*.

And yet, as progressive as *Cosmo* has been in subverting traditional gender roles by asserting female independence and sexuality, it reinscribes these roles nonetheless. One example to point to is the column entitled "Why are Men Becoming So Sensitive Lately" in "Man Manual: Cosmo for your Guy," a special section for men—presumably the readers' partners—that appeared in the September 2006 issue of the Indonesian *Cosmo*. The column itself is interesting for its suggestion that men should not expect women's position to be as it used to be, when men were more dominant (106). Yet, at the bottom right of the same page, a green box entitled "Make Him More of a Man" urges women to "give him a manly nickname," "tell him he's your hero," and "let him lead," so his masculinity would stay intact (106). Indeed, preserving traditional notions of masculinity is an ongoing theme, although rarely presented forcefully, in Indonesian *Cosmo*. Images of barechested men in its "Man Manual" section portray men with big bodies—at times with bulging muscles—in a "manly" pose that highlights their big, well-sculpted, masculine bodies. Further, in images that are set in workplaces, men are usually represented as the "boss" or as having more authority than women. In *Cosmo*, men are still considered the center around which a woman's world revolves. It is their voices, usually in testimonial form, that are used to validate *Cosmo's* attempt to reconstruct an ideal women's beauty—replacing breasts and hips with "brain and behavior," for example (Leiliyanti 2003, 79–80). This suggests that *Cosmo* can subvert traditional notions of femininity as long as men approve.

Furthermore, various ads, articles, and beauty tips in *Cosmo* contribute to the creation of gender-specific docile bodies. Feminist philosopher Sandra Bartky, in criticizing Foucault's gender neutral notion of "docile bodies," argues,

Foucault treats the body throughout as if it were one, as if the bodily experiences of men and women did not differ and as if men and women bore the same relationship to the characteristic institutions of modern life. . . . Women, like men, are subject to many of the same disciplinary practices Foucault describes. But he is blind to those disciplines that produce a modality of embodiment that is peculiarly feminine. (1990, 65)

Moreover, Bartky suggests that disciplinary practices for women are different in that they are "perpetual and exhaustive—a regulation of the body's size and contours, its appetite, posture, gesture, and general comportment in space and the appearance of each of its visible parts" (Bartky 1990, 80). Hence, using my examples from Indonesian *Cosmo*, women's bodies are disciplined in that they have to use various products from whitening cleansing milk and toner, whitening masks, or whitening cream, every night and day. And these examples, obviously requiring "discipline," are only practices for one specific part of a woman's body, their facial skin; there are numerous other examples of "care" products for other parts of a woman's face and body—eyebrows, legs, hair, breasts—to make women look beautifully feminine. The production of "feminine docile bodies," therefore, is inevitable if readers follow all beauty advice, buy advertised products, and even have sex the way the magazine instructs them.

What is interesting, however, is the ways in which *Cosmo* represents these practices not as burdens for women, but rather as expressions of women having (self) control. It is understandable that representing women as possessors of control is important and necessary, even for *Cosmo*, particularly at a time when women's equality and empowerment are acknowledged globally. Sociologist Robert Goldman, from a U.S. location, addresses the issue of control in ads:

Women are . . . advised that the path to control . . . is available via the route of pleasure. . . . At still another level of meaning, women's traditional task of controlling their figures, so long achieved by means of patriarchally enforced self-torture (girdles, corsets), has now become a supposedly pleasurable activity. However, the cultural shift in locus of control from externally motivated methods (corsets) to internally motivated methods (the "will-power" to diet and exercise) creates a new potential for self-abuse. The current scenario makes women morally accountable for making their bodies comply with an idealized image trumpeted and managed by the mass media. A new form of oppression emerges as women go to war with their recalcitrant bodies. Failure to exercise appropriate self-restraint becomes internalized as a character flaw. (1992, 111)

Goldman's point is important, for it highlights how ads invoke the notion of and attract the "liberated woman" by focusing on the issue of self-control and "internal" motivation. In the case of the Indonesian *Cosmo*, it participates in what Goldman suggests is a "new form of oppression" because, although *Cosmo* positions women as having control (over their own body), women are simultaneously told the "Six Deadly Weapons to Arouse His Love," which includes changing their image "to fit the man's taste," for example (June 2006, 146).

This representation of seemingly independent women, yet dependent on men, is not unique in the Indonesian case. Machin and Thornborrow in examining forty-four different versions of *Cosmo* across the globe pointed out how, although *Cosmo* encourages its female readers to seek pleasure and control through sex, the magazine nonetheless frames this pleasure and control as derived from pleasing men. Men and their reactions are the all important source for women's "self-image and sense of power" (Machin and Thornborrow 2003, 463). This is what literary scholar Catherine Spooner calls a "pseudo-liberated lifestyle," allowing women to fulfill their personal needs through "sex and shopping" yet simultaneously conserving more traditional notions of heterosexual femininity (2001, 299).

The problem is that this pseudo-liberated lifestyle may actually hurt women. As media critic Susan Douglas argues in "Narcissism as Liberation," when advertisers and/or women claim that these various (beauty) products are used for their own interests (not necessarily *for* men, for example), chances are problems in their lives will then be read as "personal failures," rather than contextualizing them within the larger patriarchal society (2000, 280). Applying this to my argument, I note that when women cannot climb up the corporate ladder, they blame themselves, their office clothing style, or how they have not used sex in the office the way *Cosmo* advises them, rather than questioning why women are having these problems to begin with. Put simply, this consumerism, for improving the self—from putting on lipstick to cosmetic surgeries—even when perceived as for women's own satisfaction, further empowers men.

Moreover, in *Cosmo*, women's sexuality is represented from a position that values and normalizes heterosexuality. Although the U.S. *Cosmo* does incorporate some lesbian-themed and pro-lesbian articles (Spooner 2001, 125), the magazine seems to have "the ability to make heterosexuality look like the natural and most significant referent toward which even homoerotic depictions point" (Rand 1994, 135). These attempts to be inclusive of lesbians actually create what women's studies scholar Erica Rand calls a "two-doored closet": how "*Cosmo* shows that queer visibility and queer power may not go hand in hand. When *Cosmo* opens the opaque closet door, visibility increases, but another door, perhaps stronger, locks behind it. And the benefits of increased lesbian visibility accrue primarily to *Cosmo* and to heterosexuals, not to lesbians" (1994, 129). Furthermore, Machin and Thornborrow point out that women's sexuality in *Cosmo* across the globe is represented as "the source of their power over men and of their success in the work-place" (2003, 460). As such, sexuality in this magazine is explicitly and unapologetically heterosexual.

Although women's sexuality in *Cosmo* is everywhere heterosexual, it is not articulated in the same manner throughout the globe. In Indonesia, for example, sexual acts are represented as acts between husbands and wives. This is evident from various articles that refer to male sexual partners as the readers' "husbands" (*suami*). This is not the case in the U.S. *Cosmo*. Further, Nelson and Paek, in reading 935 ads in various editions of *Cosmo* from 2002–2003 across the globe, point out how local "cultural values" and "political/economic systems" explain why "Western (or nondomestic models) are more likely to be portrayed sexually than are domestic models," except in the case of the edition of the Thai *Cosmo* where the ads were very sexualized regardless (2005, 379). This certainly is not the case in other Asian countries such as Indonesia, India, or China, where sex and sexuality are exposed to a much lesser extent.

Heterosexism, race, and skin color are also joined in the Indonesian *Cosmo* in the ways in which Caucasian white men become and appear as the desirable man for these heterosexual *Cosmo* women. An ad for hair shampoo, for example, portrays a teenage girl's excitement for a soccer game as due to the fact that she loves the Caucasian white soccer player, not the game per se. Additionally, in fashion columns, Caucasian men are represented as sexually desirable and romantically involved with Indonesian women. It seems that within the context of the transnational Indonesian *Cosmo*, the rather hazy boundaries that mark where "Americanness" ends and "Indonesianness" begins is reimagined through their (sexual) relationships. Encounters such as these are represented as "normal" and even become signifiers for the "cosmopolitanism" of these light-skinned Indonesian women. That is, their cosmopolitan status is validated through their relationship with the Caucasian white male. This in and of itself implies the ways in which whiteness is yet again represented as embodying cosmopolitanism and has more currency in this transnational setting.

It appears that these "approved" encounters between Caucasian men and Indonesian women do not invoke anxiety over the possibility of racial hybridity, unlike encounters with other races or colors. Indeed, Indo women models whose bodies are living proof of those very encounters (usually between Caucasian men and Indonesian women) are represented and evoked as the ideal of beauty. Additionally, in the "Man Manual" column in the July 2006 edition of the Indonesian *Cosmo*, four sexy bare-chested men are featured: three Caucasian American men and one African American man. Interestingly, the African American man is the only one whose gaze shies away from the camera. It is intriguing to see that in the September 2006 U.S. *Cosmo* there was a similar pattern where three Caucasian Americans were smiling at the camera, while the one African American man is represented as sleeping on his stomach, with his eyes closed. This averting of the black man's gaze in these particular examples may hint at the underlying fear of miscegenation between *Cosmo* women who in the U.S. context are predominantly white heterosexual female readers and the black man. That is, in some ways, although these dark-skinned men are allowed to appear in this magazine, their sexuality is contained by pairing them mostly with other black women, or by representing them with their gaze shying away from readers. This pattern, of course, reflects U.S. racial history.

This gender, racial, skin color, and sexuality politics of *Cosmo* necessarily provides the context for reading closely whitening ads published in the Indonesian *Cosmo*. Here I shall be employing semiotic and discourse analyses, acknowledging that "the meaning of an ad does not float on the surface just waiting to be internalized by the viewer, but is built up out of the ways that different signs are organized and related to each other, both within the ad and through external references to wider belief systems" (Jhally 2003, 153). The meanings of these ads are inevitably contextualized within the magazine within which they are published. Indeed, in magazines, ads and editorial content are inevitably intertwined. Feminist author Gloria Steinem (1990/2003), in showing how *Ms.* magazine struggled to exist despite lack of revenue from ads, pointed out that the existence of the magazine was constantly threatened because she, as editor, would not publish ads that were demeaning to women and failed to persuade potential advertisers to produce ads that highlight women's agency. Moreover, she refused to provide "complimentary" articles to please advertisers. Pleasing advertisers, to her chagrin, includes having magazines' editorial content highlight and support their advertised products (Crane 2003, 316). For example, recipes need to be written to highlight various food products advertised in the magazine in the same way fashion columns need to feature advertised clothing (Steinem 1990/2003, 223–224).

This relationship between ads and editorial content is certainly evident in *Cosmo*. Some have even noted that in the U.S. *Cosmo*, the boundary that marks where editorial content ends and advertisements begin is unclear (Case 1997). This also holds true in the case of the Indonesian *Cosmo*. For example, its July 2006 issue featured an article entitled "Does Whiter Mean Better?" Ironically, while the article itself can be considered critical in its questioning of the light-skinned beauty norm, the images accompanying this article were pictures of L'Oreal's whitening products and their model, Michelle Reis, a Hong Kong supermodel of Portuguese and Chinese descent. Consequently, the article that in some ways can be read as challenging the product advertised in the magazine is subverted by the ad itself.

THE CONSTRUCTION OF COSMOPOLITAN
WHITENESS IN SKIN-WHITENING ADS

Within its theoretical trajectories, the word "cosmopolitan" is understood to be rooted in the Greek *kosmos*, which means world, and *polites*, meaning citizen. It conveys the aura of a "citizen of the world." Eighteenth-century French philosophers used the term to highlight "an intellectual ethic, a universal humanism that transcends regional particularism" (Cheah 1998, 22). For social anthropologist Steven Vertovec and sociologist Robin Cohen, cosmopolitanism refers to "something that simultaneously: (a) transcends the seemingly exhausted nation-state model; (b) is able to mediate actions and ideals oriented both to the universal and the particular, the global and the local; (c) is culturally anti-essentialist; and (d) is capable of representing various complex repertoires of allegiance, identity and interest. In these ways, cosmopolitanism seems to offer a mode of managing cultural and political multiplicities" (2002, 4). Moreover, the way the magazine deploys the word "cosmopolitan" also falls within these theoretical trajectories insofar as the magazine seems to make meanings of cosmopolitan; as literary and cultural theorist Bruce Robbins explains it: "the word *cosmopolitan* . . . evokes the image of a privileged person: someone who can claim to be a 'citizen of the world' by virtue of independent means, expensive tastes, and a globe-trotting lifestyle" (1998, 248). Here, cosmopolitanism is framed within consumer culture to mean consuming the other's exoticized and commodified culture (Vertovec and Cohen 2002, 7). Indeed, the Indonesian *Cosmo*, in constructing an imaginary *Cosmo* woman, often suggests that readers should buy expensive gourmet cakes at elite hotel pastry shops and invites readers to travel abroad. Cosmopolitan therefore embodies the possibility of transnational mobility (the slogan's "fearless"/adventurous aspect), leisure, and pleasure through the consumption of these advertised products (the slogan's "fun" aspect), and certainly "female"-ness—the essence of *Cosmo*, a magazine for women. Even the price of *Cosmo*, Rp. 35,000 (US$4), indicates the targeted audience of upper-middle-class Indonesian women.

My close reading of skin-whitening ads published from 2006 to 2008 attests to this: these whitening ads were transnational and cosmopolitan in nature. First, almost all of the whitening ads advertised transnational brands. Except for Unilever's "local-jewel" brand, Citra, that is now also available in a few other Asian countries (and is therefore becoming transnational) and another product, Viva, all brands were transnational. Advertised brands originated in France (Dior, Biotherm, and L'Oréal), the United States (Estée Lauder and Clinique), Japan (Bioré, Kosé, Kanebo, and SK-II), South Korea (Laneige), Philippines (Skin-White), Germany (Nivea), and the Netherlands (Pond's).

The cosmopolitanism of these ads was further emphasized by featuring non-Indonesian models. In 2006–2008, unlike only a few years prior when whitening ads typically featured local, light-skinned, Indonesian women, ads featured international models such as Choi Ji Woo (a South Korean actress/celebrity) advertising the France-based "DiorSnow Pure White"; Sammi Cheng (a Hong Kong actress/singer) modeling for Japanese SK-II's "Whitening Source Skin Brightener"; Michele Reis (a Hong Kong supermodel) advertising L'Oréal Paris' "White Perfect" and "White Perfect Eye"; Ploy Chermarn (Thai actress) modeling for L'Oréal Paris' "White Perfect Eye"; Gong Li (a Chinese movie star) posing for L'Oréal Paris' "Revitalift White"; and even a few Caucasian (perhaps American) white models. Interestingly, the Caucasian white models' names are not printed in the ads. This hints at the ways in which Caucasian white models need not be qualified to represent the face of beauty, unlike the Asian white models whose celebrity status is needed to justify their presence in these ads. Moreover, because models are hired to advertise these products in several countries, they are constructed as "cosmopolitan" simply because their images travel transnationally. The meanings of these cosmopolitan models are then transferred to the product that is now embodying the model's cosmopolitanism. This process invites the reader, positioned as a cosmopolitan woman, to consume a product coded as cosmopolitan. Moreover, these ads, published in *Cosmo*, also capitalize on and rely on the cosmopolitanism of the magazine's editorial content to provide a cosmopolitan meaning to the advertised products. Using a Japanese model in these whitening ads does not suggest that they are selling or relying on Japanese-ness to sell their (at times non-Japanese) products; rather, these international models' cosmopolitanism, their ability to be popular beyond their local boundaries, as well as the meanings provided by the editorial contents of *Cosmo* magazine—representing whiteness as a desirable commodity across the globe—encode these products as cosmopolitan.

The staging of these foreign, transnational models in specific whitening ads, as well as in the editorial contents in the Indonesian *Cosmo*, hints at the ways in which whiteness is represented to have more currency in the transnational setting. First, the link between whiteness and value can be seen from an exemplary ad, the AXL whitening product. In a page divided into three columns, each column representing one product, AXL positions "antiseptic" soap in front of a pair of dumbbells (fitness equipment), "whitening" body foam in front of a woman's briefcase, and "aloe vera" soap in front of a college backpack. Here, soap (antiseptic or aloe vera) is linked to cleanliness, but the "whitening" foam is linked to "money," suggesting that for women to do well in the workplace and therefore earn more, they need to whiten their body. Second, whiteness is positioned as having more value, or currency, across the globe simply because white-skinned women (whether Indonesians or other Asians or Caucasians) are used more often than models with darker skin color both in various advertisements or to illustrate fashion columns. All of these images and ads, as a whole, suggest that white is indeed the preferred color, the color that has more currency across the globe, not just in Indonesia. In other words, traveling to Japan, Germany, or France, by way of looking at various images and reading various (particularly travel-related) articles in these magazines, the readers will see that the preferred color across these geographical locations is white.

The cosmopolitanism of these ads is also signified by their use of English; all of these ads use English, though in varying degrees. At the very least, English is used in the products' labels. The use of English in ads and in magazines functions to flatter the audience's superior status: fluency in English signifies the reader's educated and middle/upper-class position in Indonesian society. It is also used to signify that the magazine and its readers are part of the global cosmopolitan world.

If not Indonesian, why English? Remember, it was Dutch, not English, that was the colonizer's language in Indonesia. It is English, however, that has become the dominant foreign language in today's Indonesia, and in the world. Indeed, as anthropologist Niko Besnier also noted in his observation of transgender beauty pageants in Tonga, to use English is to risk being positioned as having "cosmopolitan pretensions that appear to others to seek to obliterate one's Ton-ganness" (2011, 97). And it is in English that whitening products' brands and labels are displayed in whitening ads. With only two exceptions—the French ad for "Laneige" and the Japanese ad for "Sekkisei"—all ads are in English: Bioré's "Whitening Scrub," Citra's "White Milk Bath," Clinique's "Derma White," Estée Lauder's "Cyber White," Garnier's "Light Whitening Moisturizer," L'Oréal's "White Perfect" and "Revitalift White," Menard's "Fairlucent," Nivea's "Face Sun Block Whitening Cream," Pond's "White Beauty," "White Beauty Detox," and "Complete Care Whitening," SK-II's "Whitening Source Skin Brightener" and "Whitening Source Dermdefinition," and SkinWhite's "Whitening Hand and Body Lotion." That English is used in almost all whitening labels raises the question: why does English become an appealing language to market these whitening products in a postcolonial country, and what are the consequences of such a strategy?

English, in the Indonesian context, connects this former Dutch, then Japanese, colony to an expanded world system, enhancing, if you will, its sense of cosmopolitan worldliness. When the Indonesian version of *Cosmo* was first published, the cover titles were written in the Indonesian language. The magazine's title was even written with a *K* and not a *C*, to mark its Indonesianness.

In current editions of the Indonesian *Cosmo*, however, English is used in conjunction with Indonesian for cover titles; it is English rather than Indonesian that is used for headlines in the magazine, including on the cover. At the same time, however, English still represents Western culture. Within the discourse of postcolonialism, as postcolonial theorist Ngugi Wa Thiong 'O points out, English functions as a carrier of culture and a means of spiritual subjugation (1986). This means English, as it carries the culture of a Western white empire, is embedded within the racist structure of its own society and its own color symbolism. White in the United States is not simply a color in a box of Crayola crayons. The word "white" in English represents a racist ideology at work. The word *putih*, which is the Indonesian translation of the word, cannot fully capture this. Nor does *putih cantik* invoke the cultural meaning of that which in the West is imbricated in a history of racialized color: white beauty is not *putih cantik*. This is to say that English is effective in signifying racial categories that are embedded in this language, specifically in U.S. culture. Moreover, as demonstrated in one of these whitening ads, "Pond's White Detox," non-whiteness is constructed as "toxic," as something that needs to be "detoxed." Hence in using English, a signifier for cosmopolitanism, these ads help to maintain the imperial power of the West.

However cosmopolitan these models or the language used in these magazines, white remains the dominant and desired color in these ads. The Indonesian *Cosmo*, like the U.S. *Cosmo*, circulates biased, gendered representations of skin color and race that privilege whiteness (oftentimes Caucasian white encoded as cosmopolitan white) in their magazines. Images of African Americans rarely appear in the Indonesian *Cosmo*. Even when African Americans' images appeared in the U.S. and Indonesian *Cosmo*, their numbers were significantly lower than those of Caucasians and lower in the Indonesian *Cosmo* than in U.S. *Cosmo*. For example, out of 308 pages in the August 2006 Indonesian *Cosmo*, only four pages have images of African Americans (1.5%). In comparison, out of 242 pages in the August 2006 U.S. *Cosmo*, twenty-three pages (10%) contain images of African Americans.

Significantly, the numbers are even lower for images of Asian Americans in the U.S. *Cosmo*. Indonesians or women with stereotypical Southeast Asian features rarely appear in the U.S. *Cosmo*. This condition reflects an old pattern: in analyzing thirty-eight issues of U.S. *Cosmo* from 1976–1988, Kathryn McMachon pointed out how models, "if third-world, which is not often the case, are represented in codes which signify difference as the culturally exotic. Paradoxically, actual differences between third-world or minority women and white women in the United States are denied, while racial and ethnic stereotypes are exploited" (1990, 383).

Not only African American but also dark-skinned Indonesian women rarely appear in the Indonesian *Cosmo*. There are, however, a few cases when rather dark-skinned women model for the fashion column in this magazine. In the "Sporty Chick" fashion column in the June 2006 edition of the Indonesian *Cosmo*, dark-skinned women, albeit with "European" facial features such as a pointy nose, were posed as energetic and active women. Interestingly, in the Brazil edition of *Cosmo*, there seems to be a similar phenomenon with dark-skinned women posed for "sports glossies" (Etcoff 1999, 115). However, this is not necessarily the case when "race" enters the picture. For example, in an ad for tanning lotions published in the U.S. *Cosmo*, when the now-darker-or-tanned Caucasian women are represented in a beach setting, they are represented as leisurely reclining on a beach lounge, rather than engaging in sports activities such as swimming.

Conversely, Caucasian women dominate advertisements and images that accompany editorial content in U.S. and Indonesian editions. Having Caucasian white women dominate the Indonesian *Cosmo* highlights the ways in which, within a transnational setting, not only do U.S. citizens travel elsewhere more freely compared to Indonesian citizens, but their images (mostly of Caucasian Americans) are also circulated more frequently across the globe and therefore are thought to have more value than those of Indonesians.

The circulation of these images cannot be detached from the structure that governs which images can travel—white-skinned women of various races have easier access to transnational (visual) mobility. Framed in such a way, the transnational circulation of images of white-skinned women contributes to the production of a racially saturated field of visibility (Butler 1993). This field of visibility shapes not only which images can travel, or which images have more currency in a transnational setting, but also how we make meanings of these traveling images.

LOOKING WHITE, FEELING GOOD: RACE, GENDER, AND COLOR AS AFFECTIVELY CONSTRUCTED

My argument that whiteness is cosmopolitan and transnationalized (transcending race and nation) leads us to this chapter's larger theoretical claim: gender, race, and skin color are "affectively" constructed. Cosmopolitan whiteness is more than just an embodiment of certain phenotypes and vaguely defined skin color, that is, Caucasian whites as having white skin color, big round eyes, and so on. It is *also* affectively constructed. Moreover, what is especially interesting about cosmopolitan whiteness is that anyone can be cosmopolitan and white—cosmopolitan white, that is. Anthropologist Peter van der Veer argues that "the racial distinction between natives and metropolitan has become obsolete and is replaced with the notion that anyone can be cosmopolitan, as long as one remains open, mobile, and improvising, and forgets about one's traditions" (2002, 169). Expanding on his argument, I argue that access to whiteness, in its cosmopolitan sense, and to cosmopolitanism, in its white sense, relies on one's ability to embody the affective identities constructed as cosmopolitan white. Whiteness here is not simply coded as embodying specific biological features or originating from a specific place, let alone "race," but also as involving feelings of cosmopolitanism. In this case, it is a feeling that a person is part of the global world by way of his or her engagement with the global cultural production of meanings (and not necessarily of the products themselves); Louisa Schein has termed this as "imagined cosmopolitanism" (1999, 360).

At the heart of these ads lie powerful cultural narratives of how happiness is achieved by consuming specific products. As media scholar Sut Jhally argues, "Fundamentally, advertising talks to us as individuals and addresses us about how we can become happy. The answers it provides are all oriented to the marketplace, through the purchase of goods or services" (2003, 251). Similarly, Kartajaya emphasizes that the "feel benefit," the benefit of reaching consumers' emotions and promising happiness over rational explanations, rather than the "think benefit," plays a significant role in helping consumers make their choices. As he succinctly points out, "people's actions are rooted in 'feelings'" (2004, 34). Inciting the audience's feelings and promising them happiness through the consumption of the "right" commodity is important in the advertising world.

In these whitening ads, happiness is offered via the route of whitening practices. Feminist cultural studies scholar Sara Ahmed argues, "some objects more than others embody the promise of happiness. In other words, happiness directs us to certain objects, as if they are the necessary ingredients for a good life" (2007, 127). In these skin-whitening ads, skin-whitening products become the objects necessary for a good life. Happiness is coded as cosmopolitan whiteness.

In these ads, white is embedded with positive affective qualities such as sophistication, beauty, or, as one of the whitening ads' slogans puts it, "skin of innocence." One of the mechanisms that the ads deploy to produce these positive affective meanings (such as desirability, beauty, and cosmopolitanism) of whiteness is employing certain models and organizing their faces to embody certain affects. These models, as sociologist Elizabeth Wissinger argues, become one of the nodes in the circulation of these affects (2007, 247).

The circuits of affect indeed rely on how the models perform particular affects in these ads. Advertisements function to provide the advertised products with positive (that is, desirable) affects. They do so by employing models with a particular look to deliver the product's positive affects. Simultaneously, these models are also instilled with positive affects. Ahmed argues, "to be affected by an object in a good way is also to have an orientation towards an object as being good" (2007, 124). That is, as the audience feels good looking at beautiful pictures, they will have an orientation toward these beautiful women as being good. In all of these ads, the models have white skin color, even if they are not considered Caucasian women themselves. And because as Wissinger argues in her analysis of affect circulation through a model, "affective value accrues to an image as it moves in circulation. . . . Her affective capacity increased in accordance with the number and places her image appeared" (2007, 239–240), the more these white women appear in these transnational magazines, the more they accrue affective capital. These images of "good" and beautiful white-skinned women produce positive affects about women with white skin color. This then functions as an apparatus through which the audience reads their encounter with others in their lives. As Ahmed argues, the meanings of these "stranger" others are already constructed *prior* to our encounter with them (2000). In other words, these ads help "rehearse" (Massumi 2002, 66) the audience's perceptions of the other. Hence when the audience members encounter these white-skinned women in their lives, they tend to have positive affects toward these women even when they do not know them beyond these visually and affectively constructed selves. For example, in Estée Lauder's "Cyber White" ad, the Caucasian white model is represented as a goddess-like figure. Her blonde hair is tied in the back. Her blue eyes match the blue background and the blue bottle of "Cyber White" cream. Her white face looks perfect, without any discernible pores. Here, her goddess look is deployed to capture the ultimate beauty promised by the "Cyber White" cream and to evoke a positive affect about the product. (This transfer of values can easily be seen from the white light emanating from the whitening bottle to her face.) Simultaneously, she becomes the point of positive affective identification: she looks good; she makes the reader feel good; the reader will feel good if she has her good looks and good skin, achievable by consuming the advertised cream.

What happens here is the deployment of white women's bodies to evoke a positive affect, which is similar to the ways in which, as film scholar Paul Gormley argues, black bodies are used in new-brutality Hollywood films to evoke negative affects—that is, fear—in the spectators (2005). This reminds me of theorist of colonialism Frantz Fanon's argument that the fear in the white child's body when seeing Fanon's black body, as evidenced from the white child's utterance, "Mama, see the Negro! I'm frightened!" is related to the ways in which the historico-racial schema structures how the white child *felt* about his black body (1952/1967, 111). Building on these theorists, I argue that ads are a part of the historico-racial schema that shape how we are *affect*ed by and feel certain affects toward others and ourselves. This is what I call an affective structure.

Facialization and the Affective Structure

One of the most salient features of skin-whitening ads in the Indonesian *Cosmo* is its emphasis on the model's face. All but five whitening ads (Estée Lauder's "Re-Nutriv Ultimate White Lifting Serum," Lux's "White Glamour," Nivea's "Night Whitening Milk," SkinWhite's "Whitening Hand and Body Lotion," and Viva's "White") consist of close-up images of the model's face, which fill almost the entire page. This raises the question: what affective work does this magnification of the face in whitening ads do? I will answer this question by turning once again to the "Cyber White" ad.

In the version of the "Cyber White" ad published in the June 2007 issue of the Indonesian *Cosmo*, as in other whitening ads, the face is the focal point. The face of a blonde-haired, blue-eyed, stereotypical Nordic woman fills the left side of a two-page spread. Her close-up face is magnified. A large, ice-crystal necklace fits perfectly on her smooth, white neck. The neatly arranged light blue ice bricks provide a cool aura to the ad's background. The spectator is invited to feel the "cool"-ness of the ad, of the model, and of the product through the process of a transfer of meanings among these signs (a blue bottle with a white cap, blue ice bricks, a transparent ice-crystal necklace, and the model's blue eyes). She does not smile, which is often requisite in beauty ads. This lack of a smile, however, actually adds to her innocent presence. She peers deep into the spectator's eyes with her sharp and superior look. After all, she is a goddess, or is supposed to make us recall such a mythical figure.

This return to the mythical figure of the Greek goddess is not surprising. In the visual culture world, the color white is often used as a vehicle that "takes us to the place that was held to be both the origin of Western art and its highest known form, Greek and Roman sculpture." This evocation of Greek and Roman art to endorse whiteness is racially suspect, however. This is all the more so when we know that whiteness has also been used in the visual culture world to "convey an intense physical beauty in itself" (Mirzoeff 1999, 58, 59). After all, racism works, as philosophers Gilles Deleuze and Félix Guattari argue, "by the determination of degrees of deviance in relation to the White-Man face" (1987, 178).

Moreover, in this ad the model's face is represented as surreal in its state of "flawless," poreless, ultra-white brilliance. Here, the "Cyber White" ad positions whiteness as occupying the space in between real and unreal—the virtual. Thus, the invocation of the mythological Greek goddess who looks quite modern in the ad's rendition also makes visible the realness and the unrealness of her whiteness, "Cyber White."

Cyberdiscourse, according to cyberculture scholar Susanna Paasonen, "revolves around notions of mobility and freedom in terms of identity and self-expression" (2005, 2–3). This certainly reminds us of cosmopolitanism: the sense of a globe-trotting lifestyle and the luxury of making claims about multiple (virtual) homes. In this sense, the virtual and the cosmopolitan bleed into each other. However, as some cyberculture scholars have noted, cybercitizens have often been constructed as "white" (here, white usually refers to Caucasian white) (Kolko, Nakamura, and Rodman 2000; Ebo 2001; Nakamura 2002, 2008; Paasonen 2005). Hence whiteness becomes one's access to experiencing cosmopolitanism (even if at times only virtually), and cosmopolitanism becomes one's access to experience whiteness.

Virtuality, as it reverberates with cosmopolitan whiteness, also brings to the surface the issue of real (authentic) versus unreal (inauthentic). According to the author of *Computers as Theater*, Brenda Laurel, "the adjective virtual describes things—worlds, phenomena, etc.—that look and feel like reality but lack the traditional physical substance" (1993, 8). This provides us with yet another understanding of cosmopolitan whiteness: whiteness as lacking the traditional physical substance, traditionally (and discursively) known as Caucasian whiteness. Cosmopolitan whiteness can never be "real" or authentic, nor can any race occupy an authentic white location because there has never been a "real" whiteness to begin with.

Visual studies scholar Nicholas Mirzoeff points out that adding to this lack of authenticity, virtual space is a space that "is not real but *appears* to be" (1999, 91; emphasis mine). Thus, cosmopolitan whiteness is not about claiming a form of real whiteness. Rather, it is about appearing white—these creams can make you *appear* white but cannot make you *become* a "real" white. The body can only be virtually white. The product's label, "Cyber White," therefore captures and exemplifies the cosmopolitanism of the whiteness that is being marketed in this ad. In some sense, this notion of virtuality—real but not real—bears a resemblance to postcolonial theorist Homi Bhabha's notion of colonial mimicry in which whiteness is read as white but not quite (1984).

The question, however, remains: why is the face emphasized in whitening ads? The term "face-to-face conversation" is used to signify a conversation that takes place "in person." This hints at the importance of the face in relation to one's body and its subjectivity. In his analysis of webcam sex cyber-scholar Dennis Waskul argues,

> Clearly the face occupies a supreme position in connecting or disconnecting the self with the body. One's face is the most identifiable feature of one's body and self; it is the single human physiological feature that concretely conjoins the corporeal with the self. (2002/2004, 51)

Here, the face matters because it links the body and the self. The face becomes, to build on Deleuze and Guattari's argument, a "loc[us] of resonance" (1987, 168) that allows us to make meanings out of forms of subjectivity played out in these ads. The face is a source of information through which we approximate the other's subjectivity. The wrinkled old face, the mad person's face, the evil face, the feminine face, the "Asian" face, or the beautiful face could tell us something about the person and how we would feel about them. The meanings of their faces seem so evident that we rarely question where or how these ideas arise, or why certain faces evoke particular feelings in us; that is, a beautiful face may evoke our desire or the mad person's face may incite our fear.

However, another question still remains: how are affective meanings of the model's face produced in this ad? In other words, in what way does the face evoke certain affects in others? I argue that through the organization of face, or what Deleuze and Guattari call "facialization," these skin-whitening ads function as an "abstract machine of faciality" (1987, 168) that encourages the audience to feel positive affects toward these faces. Here, I refer to an "abstract faciality machine," as Deluze and Guattari define it:

> This machine is called the faciality machine because it is the social production of face, because it performs the facialization of the entire body and all its surroundings and objects, and the landscapification of all worlds and milieus. The deterritorialization of the body implies a reterritorialization on the face; the decoding of the body implies an overcoding by the face; the collapse of corporeal coordinates or milieus implies the constitution of a landscape. The semiotic of the signifier and the subjective never operates through bodies. It is absurd to claim to relate the signifier to the body. At any rate it can be related only to a body that has already been entirely facialized. . . . Never does the face assume a prior signifier or subject. . . . That is why we have been addressing just two problems exclusively: the relation of the face to the abstract machine that produces it, and the relation of the face to the assemblages of power that require that social production. The face is a politics. (1987, 181)

Here, they suggest that the social production of face is implicated within social relations of power. It is produced at the moment of re/deterritorialization of the body and the face—here the linkage between the body and face is established: when the body can provide meanings for the face and vice versa. This process of re/deterritorialization relies on an apparatus of abstraction and facialization. This process allows the model to *affect* us in a certain way.

Moreover, if face is important in the production of affect it is also because face "is the chief site of affect" (Tomkins quoted in Thrift 2004, 61). Face has also been considered as "a colour wheel of emotions" that displays a "map of emotions" (Thrift 2004, 73–74). Hence, face can become a productive site where the audience searches for affective "clues" (Taussig 1999; Bruno quoted in Thrift 2004, 73).

In this era of Photoshop, literally everything is up for alteration, including color. Every pixel's color serves certain (affective, if not aesthetic) purposes. The easiest way to uncover the meanings of these images, according to media scholar Katherine Frith, is to alter the image of the ads and see what different meanings are produced (1997). For example, would we feel differently about the ad had the model's face been colored red and organized to look angry, that is, instead of having her lips represented as delicate, the model would show her clenched teeth to demonstrate her rage? Of course. These ads hence function as part of the faciality machine because they help the audience "rehearse" their perception of women with white skin color. Moreover, they also help maintain relations of power in which whiteness holds the supreme position. This ad feeds into the reconstruction of *her* white-skinned face as beautiful, desirable, and positive-affect generating. These are the faces we are "educated" to desire (Stoler 1995). This matters because the micro-management of desire is central to the maintenance of power (Stoler 2002). In other words, whose face we desire is always implicated in the relations of power.

I do not argue, however, that when we look at a white-skinned face, we are *always* positively *affect*ed by it. This would rob the spectators of their own agency and discount the different degrees of "intensity" (Massumi 2002, 14) that the same face may evoke in different people. This is where I agree with anthropologist and historian Ann Stoler, who argues that there is "a space for individual affect [to be] structured by power but not wholly subsumed by it" (1995, 192). After all, as Asian studies scholar Terry Kawashima has pointed out, the work of labeling others based on established racial categories involves an active visual reading (2002). That is, readers often dismiss certain parts of the body and simultaneously privilege other parts to claim that a certain figure looks "white"—in this case the Japanese anime Sailor Moon (a blonde-haired, blue-eyed, small-nosed, petite, young girl). This is what she calls a "white-privileging subject position." (Note that once again, white here is assumed to be Caucasian white.) Kawashima's article is of significance to my analysis because it convinces us of the way in which certain parts of the body (for the purposes of this chapter, the face), are privileged over other parts in order to construct the subjectivity of the other. Taking this a step further, I point out that facialization not only reveals how the face is privileged and socially produced to project various social relations of power within which this facialization process is implicated, it also shapes how we feel toward women with certain racialized and "colored" faces.

SKIN-TANNING ADS AND COSMOPOLITAN WHITENESS

In this concluding section, I would like to preempt a particular question, perhaps unnecessarily. However, it is a question that is almost always raised after I share my reading of these skin-whitening ads in conferences, seminars, or lectures: what about skin-tanning ads? Don't all of these ads simply expose the human desire to want what they don't have? My answer is no: skin-tanning ads actually perpetuate and further strengthen the notion of cosmopolitan whiteness. Hence in this conclusion, I will provide a succinct reading of these tanning ads to demonstrate how both skin-whitening ads *and* skin-tanning ads function to provide positive affects toward white-skinned women and help construct cosmopolitan whiteness.

Tanning ads published in the U.S. *Cosmo* during the months of June–August of 2006–2008 provide us with evidence that even in tanning ads, the color "tan" is advertised *without* undermining the supremacy of the Caucasian white race. Instead, these ads merely affirm positive affects toward women with white skin color and "race," and, of course, their cosmopolitan whiteness. First, unlike whitening ads, none of these tanning ads use the word blackening or browning—words that have racial connotations in the U.S. context. Rather, ads for Banana Boat and L'Oréal, for example, use the word "tan" or "bronze." "Deepest bronze," a surreal color—a color that is not often used to describe skin color—is used to describe the darkest skin tone that these women could achieve by using these tanning products. This suggests that these tanning ads do not even flirt with desires of racial transformation or desires to have black skin, let alone to *be* black.

Second, whereas none of the whitening ads hint at one's ability to take control of how white one's skin can be, these tanning ads explicitly employ the language of choice and control, an apparatus of white supremacy. Aveeno, for example, sells "moisturizer that lets you customize your color." Olay puts it even more strongly by advertising "the color you control." Hence, here the anxiety of getting too dark is eliminated because Caucasian women can control how "bronze" their skin can be. After all, as Sarita Sahay and Niva Piran found after surveying one hundred South Asian Canadian undergraduate students and one hundred Euro-Canadian undergraduate students at the University of Toronto, South Asian Canadians tend to desire skin lighter than their current color, and although Euro-Canadian women desire to have skin that is darker than their current skin color, this "darker skin" still falls within the "white-skin-color category"

(1997, 165). This demonstrates that white skin is indeed the desired norm in North America.

Third, in these ads, tanning is represented within a specific temporal (and therefore contained) context. Most of these ads, such as those for Aveeno ("you choose the shade for the perfect summer radiance for you"), Dove ("gradually builds a beautiful summer glow in just one week"), and Jergens ("a gradual healthy summer glow, just by moisturizing"), use summer as the time frame for their products. As such, tanning registers within the realm of postmodern playfulness. It invokes temporality, the changing nature of one's skin color, rather than the permanence of a desire for darker skin tone. This certainly is not the normative convention of whitening ads that do not highlight any specific time frame in their ads.

Fourth, in these tanning ads, no one is advised to "detox" their white skin color. Whereas in whitening ads we are told that white is "perfect" and that it is a signifier for beauty, in tanning ads, one is advised to simply "enhance" one's skin color. L'Oréal, for example, offers a moisturizer that functions as a "natural skin tone enhancer." This is also the case for Jergens ("natural glow face") and Banana Boat ("natural looking color"). None of these ads insult the white-skinned audience because none of these ads tell them that brown is perfect and their white skin color is toxic.

Last, some of the tanning brands in these ads suggest that tanning is a form of cosmopolitan whiteness insofar as it articulates a sense of "imperialist nostalgia"—a term coined by anthropologist Renato Rosaldo to mark the colonial's "innocent yearning" for the native's precolonial life imagined as "pure," which had been transformed by colonialism (1989). The imperialist nostalgia that haunts these ads can be seen through, for example, the Hawaiian Tropic ad, which at a glance resembles a tourism brochure. In this ad an almost fully naked woman with medium-tanned skin stands seductively displaying her curves. We only see one half of her body, positioned on the right side of the ad, occupying only one-third of the page. We see her lips, part of her nose, and one of her eyes, enough to sense that she's smiling coyly. In the background, there is a shadow of a man holding a surfboard, walking on the beach. The gender narrative in this ad is too obvious: the man is surfing; the woman is posing for the audience. The colonial narrative, however, lingers subtly in the ad's text: "Hawaiian Tropic sunscreen pampers you with its luxurious tropical moisturizers, exotic botanicals and alluring island scent. . . . With protection up to SPF 70, you can embrace the sun and fully experience the pleasures of the Tropic." Here, tanning practices become a way for white female consumers to inhabit "the exotic other" (Williamson 1986). The Tropic, with a capital T, becomes a colonial site that exists for the purpose of pampering cosmopolitan white consumers. This "going native," the glorification of the exotic other for the consumption of the white self, or imperialist nostalgia, frames cosmopolitanism as a trope of "colonial modernity"—a mode of engaging the other in the colonizing context (van der Veer 2002). While tanning products endorse rather than undermine the hegemony of whiteness, this is a particular postmodern, neoliberal, postcolonial, historical construction of whiteness that I have termed cosmopolitan whiteness. Cosmopolitan whiteness is simultaneously a form of longing for the purity of the past and of belonging to the un-rooted and re-routed world culture. Thus, although tanning ads register differently from whitening ads, they both have the same positive affective effects (that is, cosmopolitan, fun, fearless, and beautiful) toward women with white skin color. In whitening ads the English word "white" and foreign models function to infuse whiteness with a cosmopolitan flair. Skin-tanning ads in the U.S. *Cosmo*, by using the word "tanning" or "bronze" instead of "blackening," urge women to bask in the postmodern desire for playful color transformation while freeing them from the accusation of emulating blackness and hence still privileging (cosmopolitan) whiteness in its ability to travel and consume exoticized others.

In conclusion, in this chapter I point to the construction of cosmopolitan whiteness in more contemporary Indonesia. I also argue that positive affective effects toward women with white skin color are the problematic effects of a transnational women's magazine that circulates within a racially saturated field of visibility. Rather than challenging any racial hierarchies, these skin-whitening (and tanning) ads simply affirm them in much more nuanced ways. Moreover, cosmopolitan whiteness illustrates that whiteness works in hegemonic ways. That is, whiteness adapts, mutates, and co-opts new forms of whiteness to maintain its supremacy. As Ahmed points out, "freedom involves proximity to whiteness" (2007, 130). I further argue that the freedom to move transnationally involves proximity to whiteness—and this is the essence of a non-essentialist, "virtual," cosmopolitan whiteness.

5 | *Malu*

*Coloring Shame and Shaming
the Color of Beauty*

In the prior chapter, I examined advertisements for skin-whitening products in the Indonesian *Cosmo*. The analysis brings to light the transnational meanings of whiteness in the early twenty-first century. But what of the products themselves? And what are we to make of their popularity? In Indonesia, skin-whitening products are ranked highest among all revenue-generating products in the cosmetics industry. Unilever Indonesia spent IDR 97 billion ($10.4 million) in 2003 advertising just one of its Pond's skin-whitening products (Clay 2005). This sum is larger than the estimated IDR 72 billion spent on advertising anti-dandruff shampoo—the top product in the hair care industry.[1] Indonesia is not anomalous in this regard: transnational corporations such as Unilever, L'Oreal, and Shiseido have aggressively marketed their skin-whitening products throughout Asia, Africa, Europe, and America (Glenn 2008). Skin-whitening products are available worldwide in Indonesia, the Philippines,[2] Vietnam, Singapore, Malaysia, Japan, China, Korea, Hong Kong, Taiwan, India, Saudi Arabia, Brazil, Peru, Bolivia, Venezuela, Mexico, Malawi, Ivory Coast, the Gambia, Tanzania, Senegal, Mali, Togo, Ghana, Canada, and the United States. Even in countries where they have been banned for medical or political reasons, such as in South Africa,[3] Zimbabwe, Nigeria, and Kenya, skin-whitening products continue to be circulated underground (Glenn 2009, 171).

Many skin-whitening products have been deemed medically dangerous[4] because they contain illegal ingredients such as mercury or hydroquinone beyond the allowable 2 percent limit. Mercury can cause black spots, skin irritation, and in high dosages can cause brain and kidney damage, fetal problems, lung failure, and cancer; hydroquinone is known to cause skin irritation, nephropathy (kidney disease), leukemia, hepatocellular adenoma, and ochronosis (adverse pigmentation). And yet, despite warnings that the chemicals in these products may cause harm, women, who are the target market and primary consumers of these products, continue to use them.

If these products are known to be harmful, why are they so popular? I am not the first to pose this question. Existing studies on the popularity of skin-lightening creams tend to focus on the political and racial meanings of these products within the context of colonialism and/or transnationalism. In recent articles, both ethnic studies scholar Evelyn Nakano Glenn (2009) and anthropologist Jemima Pierre (2008) emphasize the need to situate the complexity of whitening practices within global racial formations. Historian Timothy Burke (1996) highlights the lack of agreement on the significance of skin-lightening practices in modern Zimbabwe where local activists and traditionalists perceive it as a sign of the "colonization of the self," while others dismiss the relationship between colonialism and skin whitening by justifying the practice as an aspect of local tradition. In discussing South Africa, where skin-lightening products have been banned since 1991, historian Lynn Thomas argues that transnationally circulated anti-racist values in twentieth-century South Africa framed skin lighteners as "immoral technologies of the self" (2009, 209). These debates are echoed throughout African-American, Mexican-American, and Asian-American communities.[5]

Other studies, as mentioned in previous chapters, focus on media representations of skin-lightening creams and, less frequently, reference biological or psychological perspectives. Nancy Etcoff, from biological and psychological perspectives, suggests that a preference for lighter-skinned women may reveal the working of a "fecundity detector" (1999, 105–106). Prospective mates detect women's fecundity by looking at their skin color believing that young and ovulating women have lighter skin. She is not oblivious, of course, to the fact that women's skin-whitening practices are also related to racism.

I offer a different approach. Although I shall also situate whitening practices within a transnational context and query their political and racial meanings, I have turned to the users themselves to ask why they use whitening creams and how they understand their meanings. What would we learn if we relied on women's representation *of themselves* as they make sense of skin-whitening practices? In 2005 I pursued this question through in-depth interviews of forty-six Indonesian women; they ranged across many occupations, and their median age was twenty-nine years.[6] Indonesia is a particularly interesting site to carry out such an exploration, with its highly variegated demography: the country claims over three hundred ethnic groups. The two cities where I conducted my interviews,

Jakarta and Balikpapan, are the most transnational in their populations: my interviewees included women with Indian, Malay, Chinese, European, and Arab backgrounds.[7] Moreover, although the focus of this chapter is on women living in Indonesia, it also attends to the ways in which women's experiences of living and traveling abroad helped shape how they felt (and managed their feelings) about their skin color. Fifteen out of these forty-six women were women with experiences of traveling or living abroad, three of whom were living in North America.[8] Interviewees came from the lower-, middle-, and upper-middle classes—the group that is the target market of these whitening creams.

The interviews led me to this proposition: that it was the urge to avoid shame and embarrassment rather than an active desire to be attractive that shaped women's decisions to practice (or not practice) skin-whitening routines. I argue that women's practice of skin whitening is a manifestation of "gendered management of affect." This gendered management of affect is also important in the maintenance of gender, racial, and global hierarchies. I came to this proposition after noting that the women in my study typically articulated their responses through various "affective vocabularies" (T. Hunter 2002, 125). One example of affective vocabulary that was often mentioned during the interviews is *malu*. *Malu* is an Indonesian term that registers not only as a mostly negative affect equivalent to "shame," but also as a positive affect.[9] For the anthropologist Clifford Geertz, *malu*, or its Balinese equivalent *lek*, can be understood as "a diffuse, usually mild, though in certain situations virtually paralyzing, nervousness before the prospect (and the fact) of social interaction, a chronic, mostly low-grade worry that one will not be able to bring it off with the required finesse" (1973, 402). In this sense, *malu* signals one's "vulnerability to interaction" (Keeler 1983, 158). Similarly, social anthropologist Johan Lindquist, drawing from the works of linguist Cliff Goddard and anthropologist Michael Peletz, points out that *malu* can be translated as "shame, embarrassment, shyness, or restraint and propriety" (2004, 487). It is culturally understood as a "moral affect" that is considered "necessary to constrain the individuated self from dangerous and asocial acts of impulse, lust, and violence" (M. Rosaldo 1983, 136). Thus *malu* could function as a "brake" that limits one's expression of his or her passion (Peletz 1996, 226). Lindquist further argues, "it is the experience of *malu*, or of being identified as someone who should be *malu*, which becomes an organizing principle for social action and the management of appearances" (2004, 488). Hence, I use *malu* here because it is an important affective term that works beyond the level of the individual, and as Lindquist points out, has the capacity to structure social encounters and feelings and to link the individual to his or her larger transnational social structures. As such, *malu* can be regarded as a negative and a productive affect, a "constraint" or a "stimulus" (M. Rosaldo 1983, 139), rather than having only negative connotations as is often the case in the Western world (Collins and Bahar 2000, 39).

Moreover, *malu*, as I will tease out throughout this chapter, is a gendered affect. Men, as Southeast Asian studies scholars Elizabeth F. Collins and Ernaldi Bahar argue, tend to "react aggressively" when managing their feelings of *malu* (2000, 48). The religious-based violence toward non-heterosexuals that occurred in the late 1990s and early 2000s in Indonesia, for example, can be understood as the behavior of religious men exercising their feelings of *malu*, according to anthropologist Tom Boellstorff (2007). Women, however, tend to be "withdrawn or avoidant" when managing their feelings of *malu* (Collins and Bahar 2000, 48). I will demonstrate how women tend to manage their feeling of *malu* about their skin color by becoming withdrawn and avoiding uninvited attentions to their skin color, as well as by performing skin-whitening practices.

There were times when the rich literature of *malu* proved insufficient to address some of the difficulties I encountered. In such instances, I turned to the feminist literature on affect and particularly on shame. For example, many of the women interviewed narrated stories highlighting specific experiences of being discriminated against because of their skin color, but when I followed up by asking how they felt about being ignored for not having lighter skin or not being considered "beautiful," many simply said "fine" (*biasa saja*) in a tone that suggested it did not matter to them. Comments such as "maybe they were just lucky" or "but we were indeed physically different from them, so [we] just accepted our fate" were also common. Feminist geographer Liz Bondi, who has written that some feelings are "unexpressed and inexpressible" was helpful here (2005, 237). Feminist philosopher Teresa Brennan provides another, but equally helpful explanation for this phenomenon:

> "Feelings" refers to the sensations that register these stimuli and thence to the senses, but feelings include something more than sensory information insofar as they suppose a unified interpretation of that information. . . . I define feelings as sensations that have found the right match in words. (2004, 5)

Applying Brennan's insight to make sense of the interviewees' comments leads me to suggest that although these women might have felt "sensations," they might not have found the "right match in words" to name them. Particularly because many women are taught to sugarcoat their feelings (Jacoby 1994/2001, 56), they might be at a loss for adequate words to articulate negative emotions.

Additionally, I identify a problem related to the "mutability," "fluidity," and "flexibility" of feelings. For example, the same affective vocabulary may mean different things in different times and cultures (Harré and Gillett 1994, 160);

indeed, the feelings themselves may change (Bondi 2005, 237). This means that during the interviews, these women might no longer harbor any particular feelings about those moments in the past; they had learned to "accept" their fates and felt "fine." Not being attentive to the fluidity and flexibility of feelings, scholars may fall into the trap of writing about feelings as "fetishized" objects of inquiry detached from their historical context (Ahmed 2004b, 32). Rather than simply drawing from theories of affect that are produced and circulated in the United States to analyze women's representation of skin whitening in Indonesia, this chapter employs *malu*, an Indonesian term, and places it in conversation with feminist theories of affect and cultural studies of emotions produced elsewhere to create a synthesis of the fields of feminist theories of affect and Indonesian theories of *malu*.

Also, with disparities between "affective vocabularies" and actual emotions one is feeling, it became necessary to look for the underlying emotions implicit in the interviewees' statements by paying attention to their body language and tone of voice, and by employing the *malu* perspective to decode the interviews. Studying affects, emotions, feelings, and senses indeed requires that we seek for "moments when affect is evident: be these smiles, laughter, jokes or hope, anger, shame and so on" (Pile 2009, 17). To understand more clearly what I mean by employing a *malu* perspective, an analogy with a "gender" perspective is helpful. Stories that women tell might not be in and of themselves gendered let alone feminist stories; yet by employing a gender perspective to decode their stories, I can make gender relations visible in *my* re-telling of their stories. Similarly, the interviewees might not necessarily have told stories of *malu* as such; however, by employing *malu* as a theoretical-emotional lens to decode these women's stories, the ways in which *malu* has been deployed in these women's lives become visible.

In what follows, I provide evidence that the "gendered management of affect" plays a significant role in perpetuating gender, racial, color, and global hierarchies and in shaping a woman's decision to practice skin-whitening routines. I present the evidence in three steps. The first step is to contextualize the preference for Indonesian white (*putih*) skin color within larger transnational and institutional structures of sexism, racism, colorism, and nationalism. The transnational movement of people to and from Indonesia has helped produce and reproduce certain feelings toward people with specific skin color. These feelings are critical in the maintenance of gender, color, and racial hierarchies transnationally. The second step demonstrates how *malu* is deployed as an "affective instrument of conformity" (Harré 1991, 45). The third step lays out how the act of covering the self with skin-whitening creams functions as a way for women to resolve their feeling of *malu* in gendered terms.

MALU IN A TRANSNATIONAL CONTEXT

What causes a person to feel *malu* to begin with? Writing from a Western perspective, psychologist Rom Harré argues that embarrassment ("the major affective instrument of conformity" (1991, 45) happens when "[o]ne has become the focus of (an apparently excessive) attention from others whose opinion one values with respect to what one has said or done, or how one appears" and that that person "has become aware that others have taken the sayings, doings or appearances in question to be abnormal" (Harré 1991, 153). Focusing on the specific context of Southeast Asia, Michelle Rosaldo argues that shame involves "the sanction of tradition, the acknowledgment of authority, the fear of mockery, . . . the anxiety associated with inadequate or morally unacceptable performance" and "embracing notions of timidity, embarrassment, awe, obedience, and respect" (1983, 141). Particularly relevant to the women interviewed in this study is the fear of mockery as a driving force for them to lighten their skin to avoid feeling *malu*.

This is best explained by using an example from the interviews: Alya, a middle-class Javanese woman born in 1973 in Jakarta and working in Balikpapan at the time of the interview, shared her childhood experiences of being called *dakko-chan* (from a Japanese term for dark-skinned African dolls). This clearly caused her to feel *malu*.

> My relatives would twist my name so it had the word "Negro" in it. At school, I was called *dakko-chan* [laughing]. So I was happy when there was someone else in the classroom who was darker than me. That meant I wouldn't be the target of their jokes.

There are various layers at work here. First, when she laughed, she turned her head away from me as if wanting to hide. This "turning away" action is body language that often suggests that a person is feeling *malu*. Even if the assumption that she feels *malu* can be applied only at the time of the interview and not necessarily to the past, it is telling that she expressed how happy she was (exposing the implicit feeling of unhappiness at being subjected to the comments) whenever there were darker-skinned people in the classroom because they drew unwanted attention away from her. She recognized that it was her dark skin color that invited attention. Moreover, these seemingly "harmless jokes" further expose the racial and color hierarchy in transnational Indonesia within which "Negro" and Japanese *dakko-chan* dolls were represented as "abnormal," and therefore a cause for *malu*. Interestingly, these racialized concepts that originated in other countries were the ones being used in this process of producing women's feelings of *malu* about themselves and their skin color.

Based on my interviews, dark-skinned people in today's Indonesia are perceived as "scary," "criminals,"[10] "smelly," "dirty," and "weird-looking." When asked about their perceptions of dark-skinned Indonesians and Africans in Indonesia, almost all of the women interviewed articulated how dark-skinned people are deemed undesirable. An example of how one of the interviewees, Ines, a 31-year-old feminist researcher in Jakarta, perceived how Africans who traveled to Indonesia (and dark-skinned people from eastern Indonesia as well) were treated, is as follows:

> Africans often get caught at the airport carrying narcotics and illegal drugs [although some of them] came here to actually do business, selling fabrics or materials made from plastics. They tend to stay in Tanah Abang, which is known as a rough neighborhood. . . . Taxi drivers sometimes won't stop to pick up African passengers. People won't walk near them. . . . Even when I came a few times to cultural events that invited diplomatic people who were referred to as "His Excellency," people still made comments [about dark-skinned diplomats]. . . . Indonesian people who are dark skinned also got that kind of treatment. . . . When a Papuan [dark-skinned Indonesian] won the Physics Olympics, people said "So, there *is* a smart Papuan. . . . " Did they think they were "jungle" people? . . . These stereotypes still exist.

Her reflexive narrative exposed the workings of color and racial ideologies in transnational Indonesia within which dark-skinned people are discriminated against. Dark-skinned people are more vulnerable to "random" checks at airports, are stereotyped as not intelligent, and are often ridiculed.

Another interviewee, Widhi (41), currently living in Balikpapan with her Australian husband, remembered her encounter with an African man in Kupang, a small town in eastern Indonesia where she grew up:

> I once dated an African. Only his teeth were white. His skin was really, really dark. This was in Kupang. He worked for X. He thought we were Filipinas. We spoke English. At first, I got scared (*ngeri*) looking at him [laughing], especially during the night. . . . I was afraid (*takut*) because I rarely saw anyone like that. He was the only one there, rare (*langka*).

What her experience revealed is that even in a relatively small town such as Kupang, transnational encounters with Africans happened and were imbued with prejudices and stereotypes about dark-skinned Africans as fearsome. I do not, however, argue that the presence of Africans in Indonesia was the *source* of negative cultural views toward dark-skinned people in Indonesia. Rather, I am hinting at the ways in which the presence of dark-skinned people, be they eastern Indonesians or Africans, help strengthen the affective structures that produce specific feelings about a particular skin color.

Although dark-skinned people of whatever nationality are often considered undesirable, the opposite is not necessarily the case with light skin color. Not all white skin color is considered desirable in the same way. In the Indonesian context, desiring white skin does not translate to desiring the skin color of those of European descent. This becomes clear in how the interviewed women answered the question, "what is your ideal skin color?" They would often say that they disliked the skin color of *bule* (a slang term used to refer to white foreigners) as well as Chinese white skin color, and that they preferred Indonesian or Japanese white skin color:

Ami (34):	I like Japanese [women's] skin color . . . Japanese [skin] is not pale. Their look is more elegant than the Chinese. I just don't like Chinese white skin.
Dian (29):	I don't like white like *bule*.[11] . . . Japanese women are so beautiful and so white, they are yellowish. I like Sundanese [Western Javanese] white; [it is] transparent.
Ina (32):	I don't like Chinese white. It looks funny. I always think of pork. It seems that [their eating pork] affects their skin. *Bule* white . . . is nice to look at. But the white is kind of reddish. So I like Indonesian white, more natural.
Vindya (22):	I like Indonesian white, which is kind of yellowish. Chinese white is too white . . . white like dead people . . . too pale.
Pingkan (25):	I think white Indonesians are different from *bule* whites. *Bule* have freckles. Indonesian white is natural. . . . I personally like Indonesians'. They [*bule*] were born white. But their white is different from our white.

What is most striking is that in specifying a particular skin color, the women use race, nation, and ethnicity to signify the skin color they prefer. The *quality* of white skin is signified by nationality and race. The whiteness of a particular skin color often becomes undesirable because of the race or nation that signifies it. This is most evident in the case of the Chinese.

The long history of discrimination against Chinese people in Indonesia seems to surface when these women discuss the ideal skin color: Chinese skin color is not preferred. Dutch colonial policies indeed produced a distinct ethnic Chinese capitalist class that has been rendered a "pariah capitalist class," occupying an "outsider" (ethnic) position in Indonesia (Sidel 2006, 19, 24, 27). Moreover, it is Chinese people's stereotypical pork-eating habit, prohibited in Islam (the predominant religion in Indonesia), that Ina gives as the reason she dislikes Chinese white skin color. Although the Chinese have light or white skin, because it is race and nation that signify skin color, their white skin color may be considered undesirable.

This reference to religion needs to be briefly clarified here. As historian Michael Laffan suggested, in the context of early-twentieth-century Indonesian nationalism, Islam indeed played a significant role in establishing a sense of identity and community. However, if Islam had not been represented at the fore of post-independence Indonesian politics, nationalism, or culture, at least until recently, it is perhaps because political manifestations of Islam were prohibited from the 1950s to the end of Soeharto's New Order in 1998 (Eliraz 2004, 72, 79). Particularly under Soeharto, mass organizations could not claim Islam and instead had to assert the state ideology, *Pancasila*, as their ideological foundation. Indeed, Islam was the target of state "repression and stigmatization" in the 1970s and 1980s. There was a shift in the 1990s, however, when Islam became popular among elite groups, including politicians and entertainers, and even became an important source of consumer-driven, "middle-class" identity. This shift was partly highlighted by Soeharto's pilgrimage to Mecca in 1991, after which he was referred to as *Haji* Soeharto.[12] It was also during this period that schoolgirls were first allowed to wear veils (head scarves)[13] to school (Heryanto 1999, 174, 175). Manifestations of Islam then continued to be more conspicuous as Muslims began to form organizations based on religion after the 1998 reform era (Eliraz 2004, 72).

Thus religion adds to the complex understanding of race, gender, and skin color in Indonesia. Nonetheless, unlike Indonesian feminist scholar Aquarini Prabasmoro (2003) who argues that the lack of a white and black dichotomy in Indonesia, even during the Dutch colonial era, is caused by the racial plurality of Indonesia, I argue that because it is race and nation that give meaning to skin color, this construction disrupts the otherwise neat racial hierarchy of white at the top and black at the bottom. This allows us to understand that in the Indonesian context, lighter skin color is *not* always better because skin color, rather than being a signifier of race, is signified by both race and nation. Lighter could only be better insofar as the race and nation that signify it is the preferred race and nation. Although there is little discernible difference between Japanese and Chinese skin color, a person may prefer Japanese white skin above Chinese white skin, for example, because of perceptions about race and nation. Interestingly, the presence of people from other countries such as Japan, China, and the United States in Indonesia has helped these women articulate the specific skin color that they prefer. Their construction of an ideal skin color is inevitably linked to national identities; it is typically constructed against people from other nations.

Although it is obvious that they do not desire the skin color of those of European descent, these women are aware that such people are considered superior and receive preferential treatment in Indonesia. This perception of whites as superior may be traced back to the Dutch colonial period. Nonetheless, a careful study of colonial society revealed that "poor whites" posed a problem and a threat to the category of European white as superior (Stoler 1995, 107). The concubinage system—free domestic and sexual service from native women—was developed as a useful arrangement to avoid such a threat (Stoler 2002, 47–48). Nonetheless, that the interviewees recognized that white foreigners received better treatment than Indonesians allowed for the possibility of reading the women's whitening practices as reflecting their desire to be treated well, and not necessarily their desire for whiteness as such.

Here, I am building on race scholar George Lipsitz's (1998/2006) notion of "possessive investment in whiteness" and Lawrence Grossberg's concept of "affective investments" to propose the notion of "affective investment in whiteness" to make visible the ways in which people such as these interviewees are emotionally invested in whiteness. Possessive investment in whiteness is the way white people are produced and socialized as whites and have a sense of material and cultural entitlement because of their being white. Affective investment, on the other hand, helps explain how "ideological relations [are] internalized and, consequently, naturalized" (Grossberg 1992, 83). Affective investment in whiteness therefore refers to how people affectively internalize and naturalize how "whiteness" (of whatever race) benefited them emotionally, economically, politically, and socially. Achieving whiteness, or becoming white through whatever means possible, including surrounding oneself with what are considered white commodities (i.e., certain education, clothing, etc.) or "looking white," therefore made sense for people as they live in a world that values whiteness.

These interviews thus exemplify how these women articulate their identity through a "felt belonging." As ethnicity and cultural studies scholars Greg Noble and Scott Poynting point out, "Belonging, and not belonging, are, of course, not simply cognitive processes of identification, but are highly charged, *affective* relations of attachment to and exclusion from particular places" (2008, 130). Feelings thus function as a mode of *subjection*, "a way in which we become both subjects and objects of power" (Secor 2007; Butler 1997a). That is, these interviewees construct their subjectivity through their feelings.

All of the women interviewed shared a story to indicate how white foreigners in Indonesia are considered "better" and receive better treatment. Here are just a couple of examples. Both comments came from women married to "non-Indonesian" white-skinned men:

Andarini (33):   Why do they always think that [my daughters] are beautiful because of their father? Don't they think the mother is also beautiful? [laughing]. They always want to know why my children are so beautiful; and they never say that their mother is beautiful. They always think that there is something else. When they see my husband, they say, "No wonder."

Widhi (41):   They always ask me where the father came from. . . . Sometimes people even thought I was their nanny [laughing].

These expressions expose the underlying assumptions that Indonesian women were considered less valuable compared to their white-skinned husbands whose "good genes" were perceived to have made their children beautiful.

As Asian studies scholar Benedict Anderson (1965/1988) has noted, one of the residues of colonial racism is that white Americans and Europeans receive preferential treatment in Indonesia. Women's studies scholar Cynthia Enloe (1989), in theorizing the existence of hierarchies of race, gender, and nations, across nations, argues that industries such as tourism rely on the working and maintenance of these hierarchies both in the host and transmitting societies. In some ways, these hierarchies are maintained for the sake of the global order.[14] I will explain this next.

Foreign workers are given many privileges in order to encourage them to feel at home and spend their dollars in Indonesia. Examples from the interviews include being seated at different lunch tables (marked as "staff only") with more menu choices compared to Indonesians at offshore mining sites, getting their requests met faster compared to Indonesian employees, or being given more expensive airline tickets so that they could fly on time when a flight was canceled while Indonesians only got their money back. Here is an example from Ira (40):

When I was staying in B. hotel [in Indonesia] and my relatives came, they were not allowed to swim. They [the staff] came right away and said that it was for members only. But when my *bule* friend came with her kid [and they were] swimming there, no one asked anything. They weren't members nor staying in the hotel. But they let them [swim]. . . . But when my relatives came with their kids, they said "members only." I even asked, "Can I pay you, can we pay you?" "Oh no, it's members only" [they said]. So it seemed that we were dirty, while *bule* were not.

This example reflects the notion of Indonesia as a good host welcoming white foreigners even over and above its own citizens, to the point of refusing Indonesians and thus making them feel "dirty" or less worthy.

Interestingly, when women moved to another country and had fewer encounters with other Indonesian women who, by way of embarrassing comments, would make them feel bad about their skin color, they felt less pressured to conform to the light-skinned norm. Ira, Andarini, and Amanda, all of whom currently reside in North America, admitted that they are less concerned about whitening practices when they are in the United States. Alya, Lily, Nia, and Lidya, who have lived abroad, in France, England, and the Netherlands, also claimed that they began to value their "tanned" skin, touted as "exotic" in these countries, once they left Indonesia. This exemplifies how "geographic mobility may be a route to different modalities of feeling" (Conradson and Latham 2007, 237). Indeed, all of the examples in this section suggest that the transnational circulations of people plays a role in producing certain feelings about specific skin colors and helps maintain hierarchies of gender, race, and color in a transnational context.

COLORING *MALU*

This chapter argues that *malu* is deployed as an affective instrument of conformity, particularly in regard to compelling a person to conform to color, race, national, and gender norms. Interestingly, the majority of women in Indonesia do not have light skin, at least not like the light skin that is on view in whitening advertisements. A light-skin norm does not really exist, if by "norm" one supposes that everyone's skin is light and one person's dark skin therefore stands out. Rather, the light-skin norm works by way of comparison. Women are compared to others or to themselves in the past. This is why the presence of others who have darker skin, such as in Alya's case, would change one's position within the skin-color hierarchy.

In the interviews, I often heard the women say that they began using skin-whitening creams after comments were addressed to them about their dark skin color. For example, Nina, born in 1977 in Kediri, who worked at a fitness center in Balikpapan at the time of the interview, admitted that in a previous job, her office mates often said to her:

"Goodness (*Aduh*), you have the darkest skin." Although I would tell them "I don't care," inside I felt like saying how dare you say that. But then I always thought about how I could look not too dark. . . . So, every time there was going to be a big meeting, I'd make sure that I whitened my skin, at least my hands, legs, and face, so that I would feel *ahem ahem* [making a sound of clearing her throat while smiling].

Here, the "big meeting" became a public space where an "audience," important in the production of shame, gathered (G. Taylor 1985, 53). It is also a point of social contact that exposes her "vulnerability to interaction" (Keeler 1983, 158), or to feel *malu*. In this case, her use of skin-whitening cream could be read as her desire to not stand out, or to conform, because to stand out would invite (undesirable) attention from other office mates. The attention was deemed undesirable because it would embarrass rather than flatter her. Interestingly, application of skin-whitening cream was intended to *avert* rather than, as commonly narrated in whitening ads, to *invite* the gaze of others. The assumption is that to be noticed for having dark skin is to be exposed to the possibility of embarrassing comments. This desire not to attract the gaze of others echoes Frantz Fanon's famous depiction of the colonial subject's plea, "I strive for anonymity, for invisibility. Look, I will accept the lot, as long as no one notices me!" (1952/1967, 116).

Nina chose to use lightening cream so that others would think well of her. Another interviewee, Ajeng (age 31), admitted that she used whitening cream so that other people would not comment that her skin was dirty (*jorok*). Women pay attention to these comments because they are "signs" that tell them whether or not they are accepted by their group. In doing so, they certainly reflect a common human desire, the "desire to have others think highly of us" as Cass Sunstein (2003, 9) has put it. The *malu* that one feels when subjected to embarrassing comments shows that one has "internalized representation of cultural demands on an individual" (Collins and Bahar 2000, 36) and that one *knows* *shame*. The feeling functions as "a type of feedback loop" that continually connects one to one's environment (Probyn 2005, 83). These women were attuned to the extent to which they had conformed to the societal norm and thus how they would fare in society.

More importantly, because light skin color is not a "norm" in Indonesia but an imaginary ideal, the practice of and comments about whitening routines are crucial in perpetuating a light-skinned norm. In Foucauldian terms, the kinds of comments the interviewees received may be regarded as "normalizing judgments," necessary for "the success of disciplinary power" (Foucault 1977/1979, 170). The very act of dropping remarks about each other's skin color normalizes light skin as desirable; it is an example of the constant "surveillance" that women carried out. Women get rewarded by receiving pleasing comments such as "you look beautiful; your skin looks lighter" and get punished by receiving embarrassing comments such as "your skin looks darker; you should . . . " (fill in the blank with various tips that women offer each other).

Offering comments about others' skin color also suggests that *malu* in the Indonesian context is "collectively shared" (Collins and Bahar 2000, 41). One's identity is linked to others' behaviors. Not surprisingly, mothers discipline their daughters, as women-friends discipline each other, as a form of caring about the other, or acting in "solidarity"[15] and preventing the other from feeling *malu*—by reminding each other, they could all avoid feeling *malu*.

Out of forty-six interviewees, only eight claimed that they had never tried any skin-whitening product. These eight women, however, admitted that they had seen other women use it and were pressed to try it but never did. However, when asked what they did every day to care for their skin, almost all admitted that there were some things they did or avoided doing because they did not want their skin to get darker. These various acts, from putting on skin-whitening cream or staying out of the sun, to choosing particular colors and outfits that would make their skin appear lighter, further perpetuates light skin as the "imaginary" norm.

The interviews reveal that skin color mattered for these women because it is one of the sources of their self-confidence. The interviewees reacted with a loss of self-esteem to comments that exposed their "abnormality."[16] In this sense, there was a specifically gendered affect produced. Some of the more common expressions of this during the interviews were:

Ina (32):	When I had to meet with many people and my skin was dark, I didn't feel confident.
Vanti (34):	Generally, women feel more confident when their skin is white.
Wati (30):	Because I was born dark-brown (*sawo matang*), I didn't have any self-confidence. So I whiten my skin to be more confident.

These kinds of statements came up over and over again, suggesting the extent to which women's self-confidence is closely linked to their skin color. An interviewee, Ira, an Indonesian-American forty-year-old stay-at-home mom, born in West Sumatra and currently living in the United States, admitted that she knew from a very young age that she was ugly and undesirable because of her dark skin color. She said:

Sometimes people would tell me, "You don't have any sex appeal. Your skin is too dark." Even guys said things like, "Why are you so black?" So, they didn't think that they would hurt you, you know. They just blurted it out in front of you, so I got used to it. Even my family, relatives, they would say, "Oh, how come you're so black, so ugly? You're a girl!" . . . I married a *bule*, but not necessarily because they're not Indonesians [and therefore considered better]. But it's the other way around. Indonesian men didn't really think I was beautiful so I had no chance with Indonesian men.

It was these comments about how ugly she was because her skin was dark, so often made to her that she got "used to" hearing them, that made her accept her place in society. She admitted that, contrary to the common assumption that women married *bule* men because they were of higher status, she came to believe that she *had to* marry a *bule* man because Indonesian men perceive her as ugly. There are a couple of points here that are noteworthy. First, although she ended up being the one who moved to the United States, it was the presence of white foreign men in Indonesia that provided her with a solution to her being perceived as undesirable by Indonesians; she learned that many of these white foreign men chose dark-skinned Indonesian women as their romantic partners. Second, and importantly, most Indonesian men do not actually always marry light-skinned Indonesian women—there are more women in Indonesia with medium/tanned skin than light skin. Yet, it was her "feeling" that played a key role here: the comments about her dark skin made her *feel malu*—she *felt* she would never be able to attract any Indonesian men. Thus, her marriage to a European American is a result of her *feelings* about her skin color.

In teasing out the gendering of *malu* based on skin color that impacts self-esteem, it is useful to take a step back and look at how women in general are positioned differently from men. Gendered socialization, as psychologists Tamara Ferguson and Heidi Eyre point out, provides an environment in which women are more likely than men to feel guilt and shame (2000, 256). Additionally, as philosopher Sandra Bartky argues, it is not that men cannot feel shame but that women are more shame-prone than men. Women bring their "general experiences," which the Swedish philosopher Ullalina Lehtinen calls "*Erfahrung*" (1998, 66), to their understanding of a particular situation, which may make them more prone to feel shame than men, even when exposed to the same situation. Thus although both men and women perform "emotion work," each gender is called on to do the work in different ways: women are asked to manage their anger while men are encouraged to express such anger (Hoschild 1983, 162–163).

There is much evidence in the interviews that women were socialized differently from men. First, from their babyhood, girls, more so than boys, received comments on their skin color and how the "right" color would make them "pretty." Second, men, unlike women, were not asked (by other people in their lives or by popular culture) to put on different kinds of makeup,[17] to cover up their otherwise "deficient" selves (Bartky 1990, 40). Whitening cream advertisements circulating in Indonesia mostly target women. The recent fad of whitening lotion for men is nonetheless marketed in gendered terms—L'Oreal, for example, launched a whitening cream for men called "White Activ," highlighting the masculine aspect of men as active beings. Moreover, the interviewees consistently revealed that men are not subjected to the same light-skinned beauty standard as women. Men can have dark skin color because, as the interviewees suggested, dark-skinned men are actually perceived as more masculine. Third, fathers, unlike mothers, were not asked to "shame" their daughters about their looks. An interviewee, Titi (47), bluntly noted the most significant person who made her feel bad about herself was her mother. Mothers are responsible for teaching their children about *malu* and for the moral standard of the family (Collins and Bahar 2000, 49–50). Fourth, taking care of their looks may not be important for men because they are not threatened by other men's appearance—unlike women, who can feel threatened by the beauty of other women because their husbands might take an additional wife or leave their spouse for a more beautiful woman. Representations of second wives as more beautiful are popular in Indonesia and certainly promote such fear.

If light-skinned beauty is desired to keep one's husband, are lesbians then immune from this light-skinned beauty norm? Although I interviewed only two women who identified themselves as lesbians, too few to draw any conclusions, it is interesting that both of these women indicated that light-skinned women are also considered more desirable than dark-skinned women in the lesbian communities that they belonged to.

COVERING *MALU*

The desire to conform, to avoid embarrassing comments, or to feel more self-confident are all adequate reasons for using whitening creams; however, I wish to add yet another perspective of *malu* to further the understanding of these practices. That is that the feeling of *malu* underpins the very act of covering one's skin with whitening cream. Various scholars have pointed out that the English word "shame" comes from "the Goth word *Scham*, which refers to covering the face" or, from the "Indo-Germanic root *kam/kem* meaning 'to cover'" (Probyn 2005, 131; Jacoby 1994/2001, 1). In addition to "cover," other scholars mentioned other expressions for feelings of *malu*, such as to "hide from that other" or to "turn away from the other's gaze."[18] Here, I once again draw from the literature of shame and put it in conversation with the literature of *malu*—after all, *malu* can be translated as "shame"—to highlight some expressions of *malu* that can be found in other cultural contexts, such as the need to hide. Being aware of these "hidden" expressions of *malu* is crucial in detecting its existence and how this feeling underpins skin-whitening practices.

When interviewees heard embarrassing comments about their dark skin color, they took note of how the skin is an important site upon which their feelings (good or bad) hinge. Managing the skin becomes necessary for the management of affect. The logic here is that if a woman *feels* "good" about her skin color, she will feel more confident in uncovering her skin. Accordingly, when she feels "bad" or ashamed about her skin color, she "resolve[s] the experience of shame" (Lindsay-Hartz, de Rivera, and Mascolo 1995, 298) by "hiding" or "covering" her skin to manage the feeling of *malu*. In a few cases, women admitted that they would rather stay home than go out when their skin was dark because, in Yasmin's (27) words, "I was embarrassed (*malu*)." Her staying home can be understood as a sign of "hiding," or in Collins and Bahar's term, "withdrawing" herself, which is a gendered manifestation of *malu*. Moreover, *malu* is understood as an emotion "that describes the failures to live up to the ideals of the nation" (Lindquist 2009, 14) or, in this case, the beauty ideal. Yasmin's feeling of *malu* can therefore be read as her recognizing how she failed to live up to the light-skinned beauty ideal. She resolved feeling *malu* by avoiding contacts with others.

In many other cases, however, *malu* is managed by covering oneself. Lindquist made the point that *malu* was the organizing emotion for the migrant women in Batam, Indonesia, to perform veiling (2009, 14). Speaking from a different context, anthropologist Lila Abu-Lughod explicates the notion of veiling and its relationship to sexual shame for women in Bedouin society: "veiling, and *hasham* generally, indicate a woman's recognition of sexuality's place in the social system and her wish to distance herself from it thus asserting her possession of 'agl, or the social sense to conform to the system's ideals" (1986, 162). Considering Abu-Lughod's argument in the Bedouin context and the fact that Indonesia is the largest Muslim nation in the world, I am not making a claim that covering as a response to *malu* is a unique feature of Muslim society, however. Indeed, as social scientist Sonja van Wichelen (2010) points out, veiling in Indonesia can be seen as a site where global consumerism, globalization, the media, and religion are negotiated. This need to cover oneself often manifests itself in the (psychological) covering of the skin with "*white*ning" cream that is perceived to have the capacity to free a person from feeling *malu*. I am extending here a notion that cultural studies scholar Elspeth Probyn articulates: "most experiences of shame make you want to disappear, to hide away and to cover yourself" (2005, 39). Yolanda's (38) succinct response when asked why she would use whitening cream indicated this: "so that when I look in the mirror I am not ashamed (*malu*) of myself." Here, the shame of the self is articulated by the very action of covering the skin with whitening cream. What I am hinting at here is this: just as popular culture often represents women taking a shower after a rape scene to signify the desire to cleanse the body and psyche, women putting skin-lightening cream on their bodies can be read as a psychological covering of their feeling *malu* about their skin color. As such, whitening practices can be (subversively) read as manifesting women's managing of that experience of *malu*.

But why, when these women feel *malu*, is it the skin that is being covered? Here, I turn to the notion of the skin as a site where the past is always made visible in the present and in the presence of others. This notion of skin as a repository of women's life stories (although as Prosser pointed out skin cannot *tell* its own story) underlies my argument that the skin and its color become a useful site through/on which women display and displace their feelings of *malu* because skin is a site where the self is "exposed" to others. It is both the public and private nature—at times what literally "borders" the private self from others/public—of the skin that allows the skin to be one of the sites through which others can "read" us and hence upon which our feelings can be (dis)articulated. I am invoking here both Harré's notion of the "body," taking it to mean specifically the skin, as a "'legible' surface from which the moral judgment can be read" (1991, 142) and Fanon's notion of "epidermalization of inferiority" (1952/1967, 13). Because the skin is (constructed to be) telling of who the person is and is a site where one's "inferiority" or one's "shame" materializes, or in Fanon's word epidermalizes, to begin with, there is a need to "manage" it to reflect what the person wants it to tell others. I am intrigued here by how skin functions similarly to shame in that it "resides on the borderline between self and other. It plays a critical role in the mediation of interpersonal closeness and distance, sensitively gauging my feelings about how close I can and want to let someone come" (Jacoby 1994/2001, 22). Hence, if *malu* surfaces on the skin and the skin may cause one to feel *malu*, it is because both the skin and *malu* function as borders between the self and others.

Certainly, not all parts of the skin are seen by others. That is why, to recall an example I mentioned earlier, Nina would whiten "at least" her face, legs, and hands prior to an important meeting. Another interviewee, Pingkan (25), explained that the face is most important for her because, "Usually people notice the face first, not other parts." Here, her whitening practices hinged on the notion of the facial skin as a site that others would "notice" and comment on. This reminds us of the discussion in the previous chapter of the importance of facialization and how face functions to represent the self. Furthermore, as cultural studies scholar Sara Ahmed has recently noted, shame is "a very bodily feeling of badness, in which one is witnessed or caught out by *others*. . . . The 'apartness' of the subject is intensified in the return of the gaze; apartness is felt in the moment of exposure to others, an exposure that is wounding" (2005, 76). Hence, it is the capacity of the skin to expose the self to others and the ways in which others may respond to that exposed skin that made the skin an important site to be "managed." But, taking it further while drawing from Harré and Fanon, I argue that the interviewees' emphasis on face and other visible parts of the skin indicate how the skin, because of its embodiment of private and public self, functions as a site upon which "moral judgments" are based. Because the skin is exposed for others to see, it grants others permission to judge people based on how "good" their skin (and therefore the person inhabiting that skin) has been. As Harré and Parrott point out, "[b]odily appearances serve as public indices of character" (1996, 50). Being judged to have "good" skin reflects on whether a person has indeed been a good, proper, and responsible woman. This reminds us of Lindquist's point of *malu* as a moral affect and its importance in the management of appearances. As a marketing executive of a whitening cream company, who agreed to talk to me on condition of anonymity, explained: "a woman proves to her family and society that she is responsible enough to take care of herself and therefore can be trusted to care for her family by using whitening cream." General expressions of negative feelings, such as "I don't feel good" (*nggak enak*), to illustrate how the interviewees felt when not using these whitening creams, were quite common. Although the line separating one's *feeling* good from a feeling of *being* good is not always sharply delineated, what is unmistakable is the quadruple equation of being good, feeling good, looking good, and having good (meaning light) skin color.

The argument here is not that the interviewees all claimed that their using skin-whitening cream was solely rooted in their feeling of *malu*. But by employing a perspective of *malu*, I allow the narrative of *malu* to become visible. That is, putting on skin-whitening cream exposed one's need to "cover" oneself with something that was (psychologically) considered un-shaming. Paradoxically, or maybe consequently, putting on whitening cream turned out to put women in a never-ending cycle of *malu*: women usually end up feeling more *malu* for using these whitening products. This is evident from the interviews: when asked the first time around if they had ever tried whitening their skin, many women said they had not. However, as I asked differently phrased questions throughout the interviews, the same women began to tell me which whitening brand they used. Riana (24), a waitress in a Balikpapan cafe, did not want to be interviewed at first because she said she never used whitening cream and hence had nothing to say. After she changed her mind, she asked me, "I told you that I didn't use whitening cream when you asked me about it the other day. How did you know I used it?" I did not, in fact, know if she had used whitening cream; but I was certain that even if she hadn't she would still have many things to share with me. Nonetheless, what so many of the interviewees suggested is that the skin-whitening practice itself needs to be covered up from public eyes (or ears), because it was considered in and of itself to be a shameful practice. Herlina, a recent high school graduate who worked at a mall in Balikpapan, commented on her friends: "They use it but they won't admit it. . . . Maybe they were afraid that they would be mocked (*diejek*) for turning white all of a sudden." Her comment further exposed the feeling of *malu* that underpins whitening practices. As Ferguson and Eyre pointed out, people tend to hide and manage their shame privately because these experiences are painful for them (2000, 254).

However, as women cover their skin with whitening cream, possibly as a psychological "covering" of *malu*, it leaves larger institutional structures of racism/colorism and (hetero)sexism unarticulated. Instead of feeling the need to "fix" these structures, women displace their feelings onto their skin and therefore feel the need to fix their skin to manage their feelings.

CONCLUSION

This chapter uses the optic of *malu* to expose how people and objects that circulate transnationally to and from Indonesia have helped structure the feeling of *malu* among Indonesian women and to show that the gendered management of affect is key to understanding women's decision to practice skin-whitening routines. This management of affect in turn maintains racial, color, gender, and global hierarchies.

Because whitening practice is in part about making the self feel good, the interviews consistently reveal that when women *feel* good about themselves, the tendency to practice lightening routines is lessened. For example, some interviewees admitted that they stopped using whitening creams because they felt secure with their husbands and in their jobs. Lily (32) said that after she was married she realized that she had her own "segment" of guys who actually liked darker-skinned women. Lidya (30) admitted that getting a prestigious job changed her desire to lighten her skin. She felt confident that with her high-paying job she did not have to submit to those time-consuming practices. Certainly, having jobs has affected Asian women's class standing and their access to modernity and globalization (Sen and Stivens 1998). Here, it seems that Lidya's economic capital provides her with a status that in turn deflects the pressure to feel bad about her skin color. If light skin becomes capital that women use to access economic capital (M. Hunter 2005), then it makes sense for Lidya to discontinue practicing skin-whitening routines when she achieved economic capital. This suggests that whitening practice in Indonesia could function as a viable means of social mobility and of articulating one's "not-low" class when other forms of expressing and embodying such a class are not available. It is important that I note here that based on these interviews desire for light skin color transcends class boundaries.

Although some women chose not to practice whitening routines because they could find other ways to make themselves feel good, only a few women resisted altogether. According to Ira:

> Because we were raised in Indonesia, we [were] groomed [to] be good wives. If you can't be a good wife because you are dark, you have to excel in something else, so I was into reading or something.

First of all, her comments reveal her observation that women in Indonesia are taught that *the* most important thing for them when they grow up is to be a wife (and a mother). One of the cultural meanings of being a good wife was, according to her, to be beautifully light skinned. However, rather than changing her skin color, she chose to compensate for her dark skin color by spending more time doing other things that would make her a good wife. (Later in the interview, however, she commented that being smart was actually seen as a disadvantage in attracting possible suitors.)

In some cases, interviewees expressed a desire to challenge the structural hierarchy. Kiki said that she had thought of writing a letter to some magazine editors, although she did not actually follow through with the idea. She said she felt angry at the magazines for perpetuating light-skin beauty ideals. When watching television with her children, she would sometimes change the channel so that her children would not be overexposed to oppressive beauty ideals. Titi said that she and her friends had seriously thought of publishing an alternative magazine. None of them was willing to give up her job, however, and so their plans never materialized. One other interviewee, Lidya, admitted that whenever someone said that *bules* were the best people in the world, she would debate them:

> I felt like I was responsible. I felt I wanted to convince them that *bules* weren't special. We don't need to think the world of them. The ugly truth is that we are the ones thinking that these ugly *bules* are superior!

Her words remind us of the power of words as a tool of resistance. A "psychology of resistance" is necessary if we are to "decolonize" "the minds and imaginations" of colonized peoples (hooks 2003, 45). Although economic compulsions, social role expectations, and beauty ideals closely interact to produce certain gendered affective tendencies, alternative imaginings are possible. It might indeed be the creative and productive recasting of national identities and gendered racial narratives that could eventually rupture this intricate and gendered management of affect.

Conclusion

Shades of Emotions in a Transnational Context

As geographer Yi-Fu Tuan articulates, "to strengthen our sense of self the past needs to be rescued and made accessible. Various devices exist to shore up the crumbling landscapes of the past" (1977, 187). This book thus asks that as we construct a transnational history of race, gender, and skin color that we make "emotions" one of these devices. This is because what one remembers reveals the ideology of emotions through which these memories are filtered. The same goes for what one represents and the stories one narrates. Emotions indeed direct not only the questions historians ask, but also the tone and content of the historical narratives they tell.

Throughout the book, I have provided fragments of history that take into account *rasa*, affect, emotion, and feeling. The previous chapters have illustrated how beauty ideals travel and help shape and shift discourses of race, gender, skin color, and beauty in Indonesia from precolonial to postcolonial times. Simultaneously, they have laid out the specific ways in which emotions are attached to representations of beauty images and that it is through these feelings that meanings of racial, gender, skin color, and beauty discourses are registered. In this concluding chapter, I pull all these chapters together and put them in a conversation with each other to explicate the theoretical implications of the book.

RESEARCHING EMOTIONS, EMOTIONS IN RESEARCH

This book makes a modest request: that we incorporate emotion and its theoretical affiliations such as *rasa*, *malu*, affect, feeling, and the senses into our research. Throughout these chapters, I have demonstrated the theoretical stake when we leave out affect theories and cultural studies of emotions as a critical lens in constructing a transnational history of race, gender, and skin color, and what can be gained when we include this lens in our analysis. That is, when we render emotion and its theoretical affiliations important in our analysis, our stories inevitably change. I offer a different route to understanding transnational construction of race, gender, and skin color and how power operates in everyday lives, one that is enabled by my engagement with affect theories and cultural studies of emotions and my contextualizing the issue within a transnational context.

By incorporating emotion into my research, in chapter one I was able to show how the formation of discourses on race, gender, skin color, and beauty in a transnational context relies on the production of *rasa*. That is, trails of stories about skin color and race in precolonial Java point us to how feelings toward certain performative subjects and events censor the kinds of history that may be revealed; for whose purposes; and to what ends. Building on the work of scholars of *rasa*, I define *rasa* as a dominant emotion felt when encountering performative events and characters that provoke our "affective trajectories" and previously "deposited memory elements" (Higgins 2007, 47). Such a concept forces us to be mindful of the ways in which emotions matter as we conduct our research. I argue that *rasa* can and has functioned as an apparatus of censorship in the production of history, and therefore knowledge. Moreover, I point out that *rasa* also functioned as an apparatus through which we sense knowledge—knowledge produced *through* and not necessarily *of* feeling. The deployment of *rasa* in my constructing precolonial history has resulted in my argument that, even prior to the period of European colonization, skin color already mattered in Indonesia and that the beauty ideal around that time was embodied by women with light skin color as is shown in the Old Javanese epic poem *Ramayana*, an adaptation of the Indian version. Certainly, during that time, skin color is not yet intersected with race. Although it is clear that various races existed, it is not clear how or whether or not racial hierarchies existed.

Moreover, by employing emotion as a device through which I tell my version of history, I point out the ways in which power operates through emotions. During the colonial period, there existed what I call "colonial emotionology." I define colonial emotionology as the ways in which ideologically permitted emotions as an articulation of the self serve the interests of the colonial empire. Colonialism hinged, in part, on Dutch women's ability to display signs of white prestige through their emotional and psychological dispositions, governed by "colonial emotionology." The representations and expressions of emotions in beauty ads during the colonial period are therefore symptomatic of the ways in which colonial ideology and power work in concert with ideologies of emotion, gender, race, and skin color.

The representation of emotions about people of different race, gender, and skin color in beauty ads and women's magazines exemplify the ways in which the construction of the Other is produced at the moment of encounter, during which "difference and antagonistic emotions" may also be produced (Haldrup, Koefoed, and Simonsen 2008, 126). In this sense, emotions then become

> ways of being and acting in relation to the world. They are inseparable from other aspects of subjectivity, such as perception, speech/talk, gestures, practices and interpretations of the surrounding world, and they primordially function at the pre-reflexive level. Emotion, then is a way of relating. It is part of the "system" that body-subjects form with others. That means that they must be intersubjectively constituted, they shape and are shaped by relations between body-subjects form with others. (Haldrup, Koefoed, and Simonsen 2008, 121)

Throughout the book, I have carefully mapped out the production of different subjectivities of whiteness in Indonesia as a result of encounters with others: from Dutch whiteness (during the Dutch colonial period), to Japanese whiteness (during Japanese occupation), to Indonesian whiteness (in post-independence Indonesia), and, lastly, to cosmopolitan whiteness (during contemporary, post-reform Indonesia).

Thinking through emotion and its theoretical affiliations also allows me to see not only how power operates in gendered terms through affect but also how people's decisions are manifestations of the ways in which they manage their feelings. I propose the term "gendered management of affects" to name the gendered ways in which emotions and affects are managed. Specifically, I point out that women's decision whether or not to practice skin-whitening routines is a reflection of how they manage their feelings of *malu* in gendered terms. I show the ways in which the maintenance of power and various forms of social, racial, gender, color, and global hierarchies during different historical periods relies on how people are controlled through affect as an apparatus of domination.

I locate affect in the space of power that is never complete or stable; it always leaves a space for intervention and rupture. As such, there are always inner contradictions and struggles. Understanding how power works through affects thus provides a possibility for challenging such power through the domain of affect. The ramification of this, then, is that to escape from the grip of power that is organized through the gendered management of affects we must find ways to resist feeling a certain way about specific things such as our skin color or beauty ideals and manage these feelings in different, oppositional ways.

This book thus functions as a call to incorporate emotion and its theoretical affiliations into our research. When we use emotion as a lens through which we sense and produce knowledge, we are able to tell different, more comprehensive stories and theories. As cultural studies scholars Jennifer Harding and Deidre Pribram point out, "emotions have played a significant role in social, political, and epistemological configurations of modernity. Indeed, knowledge production cannot be detached from emotion production, and emotional experience can be seen as a creative and insightful route to knowledge" (2004, 865). Moreover, this book also builds on feminist cultural studies scholar Sara Ahmed and Jackie Stacey's interest in understanding "how feminism has been mobilized, in particular times and places, through the deployment of different senses, feelings, concepts and thoughts" (Ahmed and Stacey 2000, 17). However, my interest lies not only in gender but also in how other categories of identity such as whiteness have also been constructed through senses and feelings. This book provides evidence for the ways in which emotions and their representations are circulated and used to construct the meanings of categories of identity such as race, gender, and skin color and how affect often functions as the blindspot in this process of gendered racial formation.

In whatever way we justify the use of senses in the knowledge production process, we must attempt to incorporate them into our research. This is because emotions have been mostly undermined in academia: "thinking emotionally" has been understood as "a source of subjectivity which clouds vision and impairs judgment while good scholarship depends on keeping one's own emotions under control and others' under wraps" (Anderson and Smith 2001, 7). Worst yet, thinking through emotions has been rendered as feminine and therefore has been devalued compared to thinking through rational thoughts.

RETHINKING RACE, GENDER, AND SKIN COLOR IN A TRANSNATIONAL CONTEXT

In tracing the formation of racial, gender, skin color, and beauty discourses from different historical periods and geographical locations, this book has demonstrated the ways in which we can use analytical tools that are locally/nationally specific in a transnational context. The construction of multiple categories of whiteness in Indonesia, for example, reveals how the concept of "race" as it has been discussed in American scholarship is both useful and problematic. That is, the multiple categories of whiteness in Indonesia inevitably trouble the contemporary American understanding of race. Indeed, "race" as a concept may not be at all useful in the Indonesian context, where discussions of race had been prohibited under Soeharto's regime with his "SARA" (Suku, Agama, Ras—Ethnicity, Religion, and Race) policy that prohibited discussions of ethnicity, religion, and race in public space such as the media. However, when intersected with other analytical tools such as emotion and space, as I've demonstrated, race becomes a useful analytical tool in a transnational context. Hence, discussing issues of subjectivity formation as an effect of ideology of emotions affords me the possibility to show that by anchoring my analysis on *rasa*, *malu*, affect theories, and cultural studies of emotion, I am able to productively use the analytical category of race in a transnational context and in the process rethink the notion of "race," i.e., as affectively constructed. Moreover, the construction of multiple categories of whiteness that follows the flows of different power relations during different historical periods shows how skin color functions as a signifier for power. In other words, the meanings of these color and racial categories reflect the dominant power structure of the time.

What needs to be highlighted from all of the previous chapters is the ways in which these affects, *rasas*, emotions, and feelings travel transnationally. From India, by way of the epic story *Ramayana*, positive *rasas* about white-skinned beauty traveled to Java (chapter one). From the Netherlands and Japan, ideas of white beauty continued to be imbued with positive emotions as demonstrated in beauty ads published in these colonial periods (chapter two). The construction of Indonesian whiteness as a result of encounters with other countries during its nation building is the focus of chapter three. Affect travels from the United States, attached to the faces of white-skinned women and Caucasian white women in skin-whitening and skin-tanning ads, circulating racial ideas of white supremacy that is cosmopolitan (chapter four). Circulation of people from and to Indonesia certainly helps configure the production and management of affect, particularly the feeling of *malu* among Indonesian women (chapter five). It is all of these attachments of emotions to differing objects and how they circulate between these signifiers that together shape the emotionscape of white beauty in transnational Indonesia. Seen as a whole, this book sketches the lay of the emotional landscape of Indonesian white beauty.

One of the theoretical implications of offering the notion of emotionscape is in emphasizing the centrality of emotions in globalization and transnationalization processes and advancing anthropologist Arjun Appadurai's notion of five -scapes. That is, in this book I point out that these transnational circulations of people and objects shape not only the financescape, mediascape, technoscape, ideoscape, and ethnoscape but also the emotionscape of globalization. When people, images, and ideas circulate transnationally, emotions that are attached to these subjects/objects also travel with them and change the emotionscape of these transnational spaces. Indeed, there are emotional reasons behind these transnational movements; experiences of encountering others in a transnational context are also affective. Moreover, by theorizing the notion of emotionscape, I demonstrate that affective meanings of certain spaces help configure the formation of gendered and racialized subjectivity. This book thus makes visible not only the centrality of affective production in the construction of space and race, but also the range of feelings that a certain place is filled with and how they are employed to justify gender, racial, spatial, and national hierarchies. Additionally, the theoretical contribution of emotionscape specifically in media studies is a call to critically examine the emotional background of ads: how emotions are represented and circulated in visual culture, and for what (affective) purposes.

Theorizing race, gender, and skin color in a transnational context through the lens of affects also provides me with a theoretical venue to argue that race, gender, and skin color are affectively, virtually, and transnationally constructed. I also point to the construction of cosmopolitan whiteness: a signifier without a racialized, signified body. Cosmopolitan whiteness can and has been modeled by women with different racial and national backgrounds. By pointing out the construction of cosmopolitan whiteness, I suggest that there isn't any one race that occupies an authentic cosmopolitan white location because there has never been a "real" whiteness to begin with: whiteness is a virtual quality, neither real nor unreal.

This transnational lens that I use to understand the construction of an ideal beauty in Indonesia not only allows me to point to the emergence of multiple categories of whiteness but also affords me a way to escape from the binary route that leads to the argument that a specific beauty culture is rooted either in a national/traditional practice (Leung, Lam, and Sze 2001) or in desires to mimic American and European whiteness. Thus, by using a transnational perspective, I point to the dominant discourses that an Indonesian white beauty ideal is responding to: Indonesian white beauty is a modern/contemporary/postcolonial construction of an ideal of women's beauty that emerges out of a long process of encounters with and resistance to Dutch colonialism, Japanese occupation, and American cultural hegemony and attempts to strategically represent and position Indonesian women within this global racial hierarchy.

Nonetheless, throughout this process I also reveal the normalization of white skin color as the standard of beauty across different nations. That is, Indonesian white beauty disrupts, challenges, but simultaneously reaffirms white as the superior and most desirable color across nations. Indonesian whiteness can be understood as how Indonesians interpret whiteness in their own sense. Indonesian scholar Mona Lohanda noted that "the nationalists . . . were not the interpreters of the indigenous traditions, but the importers of a foreign intellectual and political ideas, being familiar with the western style of thinking" (2002, 12). As such, the construction of Indonesian whiteness might sit well with the postcolonial critic Homi Bhabha's argument of "colonial mimicry" (the ways in which colonized people strive to be "almost the same, *but not quite*") and as such the position of the colonized merely strengthens the position of the colonizer (1984, 126). Hence, while it is true that the majority and dominant people in Indonesia are not Caucasian and that the dominant beauty discourse in Indonesia is one that values a specifically Indonesian whiteness or cosmopolitan whiteness, one should not easily dismiss the relationship between Indonesia white beauty and global "white supremacy." The particular social formation of Indonesia provides us with a different story, a different way of understanding and theorizing affect and power and social categories of identity. To contextualize this issue within a colonial and transnational context is to provide an understanding of how representation of emotion operates as an articulation of power, particularly in regard to race and gender issues, in a transnational space.

That people and objects constantly travel across national boundaries necessitates that we investigate the meanings of skin color beyond our national border. As critical theorists Donaldo Macedo and Panayota Gounari point out, "[p]ower is no longer tied to any geographical location and is not contained within nation-states. On the contrary, power is extraterritorial; it flows" (2006, 14). We therefore need to follow this flow of power beyond a single nation-state to thoroughly understand the power of whiteness. It is my hope that future research incorporates not only analyses of the physical, political, social, and visual backgrounds but also the emotional environment of processes of transnationalization, globalization, and identity formation.

NOTES

Introduction

1 This anxiety of "being seen," because it may lead to surveillance, bears a similar emotional resemblance to the colonial Indonesian period when the Dutch forbade the natives to see the colonizers especially when the colonizers were watching the colonized. At that time, a telescope became a powerful optical tool that would allow someone to "get inside to hide and watch" (Mrázek 1999, 39).

2 In the postmodern world that is "figural and sensory," senses are constructed as "both sensation and meaning," "a medium and a message" (Rodaway 1994, 7, 25–56).

3 Indonesian is touted as one of the "simplest languages in the world," not having any "tenses, grammatical gender, tones, or articles, and its few plurals are made by simply repeating the word" (Mirpuri 1990, 86).

4 Malay is a language that was first circulated through trade routes; it is still spoken in Malaysia, albeit in different forms (due to different colonial histories in these two countries), providing evidence for its transnational circulations (Sneddon 2003, 7–9, 11). Moreover, the presence of Arabs in the archipelago also imprinted its influence in Malay. Arabic constitutes approximately fifteen percent of Malay vocabularies (J. Taylor 2003, 105–106).

5 This was a common language used in the sixth- to twelfth-century Sriwijayan (Sumatra) empire (Rafferty 1984, 247).

6 In the 1920s–1930s, it was Dutch, Malay, and local dialects that were the languages of debate (Sutherland 1979, 107).

7 Indonesia has three time zones: Indonesia Bagian Barat (Western Indonesia), Indonesia Bagian Tengah (Central Indonesia), and Indonesia Bagian Timur (Eastern Indonesia). Hence, "Western Indonesia" refers to islands located within the first time zone such as Java and Sumatra.

8 Most of these workers came from Japan (3,500), South Korea (1,900), the United States, Australia, England, India, Canada, Malaysia, and China (about 1,500 each). (http://www.nakertrans.go.id/pusdatinnaker/tka/TKA_WNegara%202004.htm http://www.nakertrans.go.id/pusdatinnaker/tka/TKA_Jab2004.htm and http://www.nakertrans.go.id/pusdatinnaker/tka/TKA_Jab%202004.htm.) This number does not include families accompanying these workers, tourists, students, unemployed, and other undocumented workers and foreigners in Indonesia.

9 Brian Massumi defines emotion as "qualified intensity, the conventional, consensual point of insertion of intensity into semantically and semiotically formed progressions, into narrativizable action-reaction circuits, into function and meaning. It is intensity owned and recognized" (2002, 28).

Chapter 1: *Rasa*, Race, and *Ramayana*

1 "Transnational" is put in scare quotes here to highlight the limitations of the term: circulations of people, images, and ideas prior to the formation of the nation-state or beyond the "nation-state" framework could elude us unless we expand our understanding of transnationalism.
2 This is the version that most scholars in the field use. See Helen Creese (2004).
3 Raksasi is the feminine form of raksasa, meaning monster, demon, or huge creature.
4 In places such as Melanesia and New Guinea, people have two different moon gods: "one for the waxing who was bright, good and lucky, and one for the waning who was dark, bad and unlucky" (Cashford 2003, 127). Hence whereas the dark moon signifies anxiety and trouble and a dark sun represents a bad omen, the bright moon represents happiness and the bright sun stands for good things (Pathak 1968, 134, 140).
5 It is important to acknowledge that during this period, a few of the gods were constructed as dark skinned, revealing the complex nature of skin color at this time. Interestingly, although both the god Shiva and his wife goddess Kali are represented by the color black, it is the female goddess Kali who wears a necklace made of skulls and is considered to reveal the "'black' dimension of Time," while Shiva who is also referred to as Kala, meaning the "Black One," represents eternity, exposing the gendered nature of color (Cashford 2003, 66).

Chapter 2: Rooting and Routing Whiteness in Colonial Indonesia

1 Based on fieldwork in the 1950s in Modjokuto, a small town in east-central Java with a population of 20,000 people (18,000 were Javanese, 1,800 Chinese, and the rest Arabs, Indians, and other minorities), Geertz (1960) offered three categories of Javanese religious practice: *abangan*, *santri*, and *priyayi*.
2 *Abangan* here refers to "religious tradition [that is] made up primarily of the ritual feast called the *slametan*, an extensive and intricate complex of spirit beliefs, and a whole set of theories and practices of curing, sorcery, and magic" (Geertz 1960, 5, 127).
3 Some would argue that Islam was successfully disseminated in Java because Islam was made "compatible with [people's] own views" (Robson 1981, 5).
4 People who were categorized as *santri* tended to pay more attention to Islamic doctrine and the "moral and social interpretation of it" (Geertz 1960, 127).

5 The two largest Muslim organizations in Indonesia are Nahdlatul Ulama (NU) and Muhammadiyah (Mulkhan 2002, 216).

6 Around this same time (mid-nineteenth and early twentieth centuries), Chinese women also began to migrate to Southeast Asia (Sidel 2006, 23). These waves of migration might perhaps be understood as a result of fare reduction in transportation (Mulyana 2005, 86).

7 Not surprisingly, most people in academia, at least after 1965, came from families who had aristocratic, business, or civil servant backgrounds (MacDougall quoted in Farid 2005, 169–170).

8 *Tanam Paksa* was a sharecropping system that benefited the colonial government.

9 In 1920, statistics indicated that there were four million people, both men and women, who could read (Locher-Scholten 2000, 19).

10 For a history of newspapers and advertising in newspapers from 1870–1915, see Bedjo Riyanto (2000).

11 Based on 1930 data, women made up 25 percent of workers at sugar plantations and 45 percent of workers at other European plantations in Java (Locher-Scholten 2000, 51).

Chapter 3: Indonesian White Beauty

1 See Rudolf Mrázek (1999); Wolfgang Schivelbusch (1995); Benedict Anderson (1990); and Vera Mackie(1995).

2 An article published in *Wanita* in 1960 suggested that bleaching cream could be used to whiten black spots from acne.

3 It is worthy of note that analysis of class was suppressed particularly because Soeharto's family and cronies (including some key Chinese-Indonesian entrepreneurs) constituted a powerful capitalist group, exploiting Indonesians across the archipelago for their own profit through "forceful appropriation," rather than merely capital investments (Vickers 2005, 185–186).

4 This policy is known as *Surat Izin Usaha Penerbitan Pers* (SIUPP).

5 This narrative that proximity to (or being in) certain places could yield specific affective results such as happiness has been used in migration narratives as well. That is, although many people do not necessarily migrate to America or Europe and instead migrate to third world countries, narratives of migration are mostly dominated by migration stories to Europe and America. This is because these are the places to which positive affects such as feeling free and happy are usually represented to be attached.

6 Karen Strassler, who pointed out that Chinese-Indonesians also take part in visually imagining the nation, noted that Chinese photographers framed the "authentic" Indonesia with a tint of "romantic nostalgia," as "lush tropical landscapes and the picturesquely rendered lives of the rural poor" (2008, 428).

7 This trend shifts again after 2000.

Chapter 4: *Cosmopolitan* Whiteness

1 Whitening ads are published throughout the year in the Indonesian *Cosmo*. For this chapter, I focus on thirty-four whitening ads published in the summer months (June, July, and August) of 2006, 2007, and 2008. I also provide an analysis of a total of nine tanning ads published in the U.S. *Cosmo* during the same months and years.

2 Allen Pope was a U.S. air force pilot whose aircraft was shot down while flying over eastern Indonesia as part of this covert operation that supported rebels in Indonesia. He was then captured by Indonesians on May 19, 1958 and sentenced to death. After pressures from the U.S. administration, the Indonesian government let him go (Kahin and Kahin 1995, 182).

Chapter 5: *Malu*

1 From 2007 data, http://www.asiamedia.ucla.edu/article.asp?parentid=70144 (accessed August 25, 2009).

2 More than two million skin-lightening products were sold per year in the Philippines. See Joanne Rondilla (2009, 63).

3 Before skin lighteners were banned in 1991 in South Africa, skin-lightening products reaped 70 million South African rand (US$27 million). See Lynn Thomas (2009, 188).

4 Whitening products come in different forms: creams, pills, body and facial soaps, "papaya" soaps, moisturizers, facial cleansers, deodorants, sunblocks, lamb placenta, prescribed drugs, and injections. Most of the interviewees used whitening soaps, lotions, and moisturizers, which they applied twice daily—Pond's and Citra were the two most popular brands among my interviewees. These creams, according to the dermatologist whom I interviewed, are usually not effective because they contain 2% or less of hydroquinone—5% hydroquinone is required to be effective. To buy products with a higher level of hydroquinone, Indonesian women have to go to dermatologists, beauty salons, or the underground markets.

5 See Ronald Hall (1995); Kathy Peiss (1998); Joanne Rondilla and Paul Spickard (2007); and Margaret Hunter (2005).

6 I used snowball and random methods. I chose Jakarta because it is the most developed, most populated, and most transnational city in Indonesia. I also included Balikpapan, a city in the island of Kalimantan—to avoid a "Java-centric" research. Balikpapan has the highest number of foreign workers in Kalimantan Island.

7 Although the women I interviewed lived in Jakarta and Balikpapan, they came from various cities on the island of Java (Bandung, Brebes, Cianjur, Gombong, Indramayu, Jakarta, Kediri, Pekalongan, Purwodadi, Semarang, Sidoarjo, Solo, Sukanagalih, Surabaya), Kalimantan Island (Balikpapan, Banjarmasin, Pulau Bulu, Tarakan), Sumatra Island (Medan, Padang, Palembang), Bali, and various other

islands from the eastern part of Indonesia (Maluku, Sumba, Ternate); and one was born in Portugal. The interviewees included women with Indian, Malay, Chinese, European, and Arab backgrounds. Their occupations were: engineers, domestic workers, homemakers, sales associates, herb beverage (*jamu*) sellers, owners of small convenience stores, researchers, live-in nannies, preschool teachers, bookstore attendants, gas station attendants, waitresses, students, foreign language teachers, entrepreneurs, and event organizers. A few occupied managerial level positions at transnational corporations while others were unemployed high school graduates. One of the women was illiterate; several had not graduated from elementary school; many were high school graduates; some had completed four years of college education and even attained master's degrees. Most of these women were heterosexual; only two women identified themselves as lesbians. Almost everyone was abled-bodied, except for one woman who was partially blind. At the time of the interviews, these women were in their twenties (24 people), thirties (18 people), forties (1 person), fifties (2 people), and eighties (1 person). The median age was twenty-nine.

8 I put these women's narratives in conversation with each other, rather than grouping them based on the city where they lived. I did so to demonstrate the similarities and linkages of these women's stories living in different cities and to show that skin-whitening practices are found across various geographical locations among women in Indonesia, and to show how their feelings toward their skin color changed once they moved abroad. As such, I do not essentialize them—I note and recognize their differences when appropriate.

9 See Eve Sedgwick and Adam Frank (1995), on the transformative aspect of shame.

10 In Indonesia, criminals are most often represented as lower class. See James Siegel (1998).

11 *Bule* (pronounced boo-lay) is a slang term for foreigner, particularly a foreigner of white European descent. My subjects frequently used this term and I have retained it here to convey their voice.

12 It should be noted that the title *haji* (Muslim-man pilgrim) once demonstrated one's economic status because *haji* used to be associated with a "rich man" (Geertz 1960, 134). That religion is intertwined with status is not a new phenomenon. This can be seen, for example, from the fact that because migrants from Hadrami in the past usually were merchants and had some economic power, their economic positions provided them with religious status (Eliraz 2004, 49–50). At that time, Arabs from Hadramaut were perceived as upper class and the elite of the Islamic community. Also, because they tended to intermarry with local women (female immigration was limited at that time), they were not seen as outsiders within the community.

13 Around this time, there was a sudden boom in the Muslim women's clothing industry. Interestingly, designers of this clothing admitted that it was the "international" or "Western" world rather than the Arab world that became their sources of inspiration (Heryanto 1999, 175).

14 Indonesian feminist Julia Suryakusuma points out that Indonesian women migrant workers' representation as timid or *malu* has been exploited as one of their "selling points." See Suryakusuma (2004, 313).

15 To understand how *malu* is linked to "social harmony and group solidarity," see Collins and Bahar (2000, 42).

16 In the American context, Sandra Bartky, citing John Rawls, pointed out, "shame is an emotion felt upon the loss of self-esteem." See her *Femininity and Domination*, 1990, 87.

17 In South Korea men have begun to use whitening cream.

18 See Sara Ahmed (2005, 75); and Janice Lindsay-Hartz, Joseph de Rivera, and Michael Mascolo (1995, 295).

REFERENCES

Abbi, Kumool. 2002. "Myth of the Sun and the Moon." In *Signification in Language and Culture*, edited by Harjeet Singh Gill, 509–535. Shimla: Indian Institute of Advanced Study.

Abdullah, Taufik. 2001. *Nasionalisme dan Sejarah*. Bandung: Satya Historika.

Abidin, Wikrama. 2005. *Politik Hukum Pers Indonesia*. Jakarta: Grasindo.

Abu-Lughod, Lila. 1986. *Veiled Sentiments: Honor and Poetry in a Bedouin Society*. Berkeley: University of California Press.

Adesh, Hari. 1992. "Various Ramayanas." In *Ramayana: Its Universal Appeal and Global Role*, edited by Lallan Prasad Vyas, 9–15. Delhi: Har-Anand Publications.

Ahmed, Sara. 2010. *The Promise of Happiness*. Durham, NC: Duke University Press.

———. 2007. "Multiculturalism and the Promise of Happiness." *New Formations* 63: 121–137.

———. 2005. "The Politics of Bad Feeling." *Australian Critical Race and Whiteness Studies Association Journal* 1: 72–85.

———. 2004a. "Affective Economies." *Social Text* 22, no. 2: 117–139.

———. 2004b. *The Cultural Politics of Emotion*. Edinburgh: Edinburgh University Press.

———. 2000. *Strange Encounters: Embodied Others in Post-Coloniality*. London: Routledge.

Ahmed, Sara, and Jackie Stacey, eds. 2000. *Transformations: Thinking through Feminism*. London: Routledge.

Ambardekar, R. 1979. *Rasa Structure of the Meghaduta (A Doctoral Work)*. Bombay, India: Adreesh Prakashan.

Anderson, Benedict. 1983/2006. *Imagined Communities: Reflections on the Origin and Spread of Nationalism*. London: Verso.

———. 1990. *Language and Power: Exploring Political Cultures in Indonesia*. Ithaca, NY: Cornell University Press.

———. 1965/1988. *Mythology and the Tolerance of the Javanese*. Ithaca, NY: Cornell University Southeast Asia Program Publications.

Anderson, Kay, and Susan Smith. 2001. "Editorial: Emotional Geographies." *Transactions of the Institute of British Geographers* 26, no. 1: 7–10.

Anshory, Irfan. 2004. "Asal Usul Nama Indonesia" *Pikiran Rakyat: pikiran-rakyat.com*. Aug. 16, 2004. Nov. 10, 2006. <http://www.pikiran-rakyat.com/cetak/0804/16/0802.htm>

Appadurai, Arjun. 2003. "Sovereignty without Territoriality: Notes for a Postnational Geography." In *The Anthropology of Space and Place: Locating Culture*, edited by Setha M. Low and Denise Lawrence-Zuniga, 337–349. Malden, MA: Blackwell.

———. 1996. *Modernity at Large: Cultural Dimensions of Globalization*. Minneapolis: University of Minnesota Press.

Asher, Catherine, and Cynthia Talbot. 2006. *India before Europe*. Cambridge: Cambridge University Press.

Ashikari, Mikiko. 2005. "Cultivating Japanese Whiteness: The 'Whitening' Cosmetics Boom and the Japanese Identity." *Journal of Material Culture* 10, no. 1: 73–95.

Bandem, I Made. 1992. "Source of Delight and Ethical Precepts in Bali." In *Ramayana: Its Universal Appeal and Global Role*, edited by Lallan Prasad Vyas, 59–71. Delhi: Har-Anand Publications.

Barnes, Natasha. 2000. "Face of the Nation: Race, Nationalisms, and Identities in Jamaican Beauty Pageants." In *The Gender and Consumer Culture Reader*, edited by Jennifer Scanlon, 355–371. New York: New York University Press.

Bartky, Sandra. 1990. *Femininity and Domination*. New York: Routledge.

Bashford, Alison, and Philippa Levine. 2010. *The Oxford Handbook of the History of Eugenics*. Oxford: Oxford University Press.

Benamou, Marc. 2010. *Rasa: Affect and Intuition in Javanese Musical Aesthetics*. Oxford: Oxford University Press.

Berg, Lawrence, and Robin Kearns. 1996. "Naming as Norming: 'Race,' Gender, and the Ideological Politics of Naming Places in Aotearoa/New Zealand." *Environment and Planning D: Society and Space* 14: 99–122.

Besnier, Niko. 2011. *On the Edge of the Global: Modern Anxieties in a Pacific Island Nation*. Stanford, CA: Stanford University Press.

Bhabha, Homi. 1984. "Of Mimicry and Man: The Ambivalence of Colonial Discourse." *October* 28: 125–133.

Bhat, G. K. 1984. *Rasa Theory and Allied Problems*. Baroda, India: University of Baroda Press.

Blank, Jonah. 1992. *Arrow of the Blue-Skinned God: Retracing Ramayana through India*. New York: Image Books.

Blussé, Léonard. 1986. *Strange Company: Chinese Settlers, Mestizo Women, and the Dutch in VOC Batavia*. Dordrecht: Foris.

Boellstorff, Tom. 2007. *A Coincidence of Desires: Anthropology, Queer Studies, Indonesia*. Durham, NC: Duke University Press.

Bondi, Liz. 2005. "The Place of Emotions in Research: From Partitioning Emotion and Reason to the Emotional Dynamics of Research Relationships." In *Emotional Geographies*, edited by Liz Bondi, Joyce Davidson, and Mick Smith, 228–246. Aldershot, UK: Ashgate.

Bonnett, Alastair. 2002. "A White World? Whiteness and the Meaning of Modernity in Latin America and Japan." In *Working Through Whiteness: International Perspectives*, edited by Cynthia Levine-Rasky, 69–106. Albany: SUNY Press.

Bordo, Susan. 1997. "'Material Girl': The Effacements of Postmodern Culture." In *The Gender/Sexuality Reader*, edited by Roger Lancaster and Micaela Di Leonardo, 335–358. New York: Routledge.

Bose, Mandakranta, ed. 2004. *The Ramayana Revisited*. Oxford: Oxford University Press.

Brennan, Teresa. 2004. *The Transmission of Affect*. Ithaca, NY: Cornell University Press.

Brown, Michael. 2006. "A Geographer Reads *Geography Club*: Spatial Metaphor and Metonym in Textual/Sexual Space." *Cultural Geographies* 13: 313–339.

Bruno, Giuliana. 2002. *Atlas of Emotion: Journeys in Art, Architecture, and Film*. New York: Verso.

Burke, Timothy. 1996. *Lifebuoy Men, Lux Women: Commodification, Consumption, and Cleanliness in Modern Zimbabwe*. Durham, NC: Duke University Press.

Butler, Judith. 1997a. *The Psychic Life of Power: Theories in Subjection*. Stanford, CA: Stanford University Press.

———. 1997b. *Excitable Speech: A Politics of the Performative*. New York: Routledge.

———. 1993. "Endangered/Endangering: Schematic Racism and White Paranoia." In *Reading Rodney King: Reading Urban Uprising*, edited by Robert Gooding-Williams, 15–22. New York: Routledge.

———. 1990. *Gender Trouble: Feminism and the Subversion of Identity*. New York: Routledge.

Calhoun, Lindsay. 2005. "'Will the Real Slim Shady Please Stand Up?' Masking Whiteness, Encoding Hegemonic Masculinity in Eminem's *Marshall Mathers* LP." *The Howard Journal of Communications* 16: 267–294.

Carr, David. 2002. "Romance, in *Cosmo*'s World, Is Translated in Many Ways." *New York Times*. May 26, 2002. http://tiny.cc/t12ks (accessed August 16, 2010).

Case, Tony. 1997. "Fearless Female Takes Over from 'Cosmo' Girl." *Advertising Age* 68: 43.

Cashford, Jules. 2003. *The Moon: Myth and Image*. New York: Four Walls Eight Windows.

Chancer, Lynn. 1998. *Reconcilable Differences: Confronting Beauty, Pornography, and the Future of Feminism*. Berkeley: University of California Press.

Chang, Jui-Shan. 2004. "Refashioning Womanhood in 1990s Taiwan: An Analysis of the Taiwanese Edition of *Cosmopolitan* Magazine." *Modern China* 30, no. 3: 361–397.

Chatterji, B. R. 1967. *History of Indonesia: Early and Medieval*. Meerut, India: Meenakshi Prakashan.

Cheah, Peng. 1998. "Introduction Part II: The Cosmopolitical—Today." In *Cosmopolitics: Thinking and Feeling Beyond the Nation*, edited by Peng Cheah and Bruce Robbins, 20–44. Minneapolis: University of Minnesota Press.

Clay, Jason W. 2005. *Exploring the Links between International Business and Poverty Reduction: A Case Study of Unilever in Indonesia*. London: Oxfam GB, Novib Oxfam Netherlands, and Unilever.

Clifford, James. 1997. *Routes: Travel and Translation in the Late Twentieth Century*. Cambridge, MA: Harvard University Press.

Clough, Patricia, and Jean Hayley, eds. 2007. *The Affective Turn: Theorizing the Social*. Durham, NC: Duke University Press.

Coedès, George. 1968. *The Indianized States of Southeast Asia*. Edited by Walter F. Vella. Translated by Susan Cowing. Honolulu: East-West Center.

Cohen, Philip. 1994. *Home Rules: Some Reflections on Racism and Nationalism in Everyday Life*. Essex: University of East London.

Collins, Elizabeth F., and Ernaldi Bahar. 2000. "To Know Shame: *Malu* and Its Uses in Malay Societies." *Crossroads: An Interdisciplinary Journal of Southeast Asian Studies* 14, no. 1: 35–69.

Colombijn, Freek. 2000. "The Emergence of 'Racial' Boundaries in Nineteenth-Century Towns in Sumatra (Indonesia)." In *Metropolitan Ethnic Culture: Maintenance and Interaction*, edited by China Urban Anthropology Association, 44–55. Beijing: Academy Press.

Conradson, David, and Alan Latham. 2007. "The Affective Possibilities of London: Antipodean Transnationals and the Overseas Experience." *Mobilities* 2, no. 2: 231–254.

Cooper, Frederick, and Ann Stoler, eds. 1997. *Tensions of Empire: Colonial Cultures in a Bourgeois World*. Berkeley: University of California.

Cosgrove, Denis. 1984. *Social Formation and Symbolic Landscape*. London: Croom Helm.

Coté, Joost. 2001. "Being White in Tropical Asia: Racial Discourses in the Dutch and Australian Colonies at the Turn of the Twentieth Century." *Itinerario* 25: 112–135.

Crane, Diana. 2003. "Gender and Hegemony in Fashion Magazines: Women's Interpretations of Fashion Photographs." In *Gender, Race, and Class in Media*, 2nd ed., edited by Gail Dines and Jean Humez, 314–332. Thousand Oaks, CA: Sage.

Creighton, Millie. 1997. "Soto Others and Uchi Others: Imaging Racial Diversity, Imagining Homogeneous Japan." In *Japan's Minorities: The Illusion of Homogeneity*, edited by Michael Weiner, 211–238. London: Routledge.

Creese, Helen. 2004. *Women of the Kakawin World: Marriage and Sexuality in the Indic Courts of Java and Bali*. New York: M. E. Sharpe.

Daniels, Stephen. 1993. *Fields of Vision: Landscape Imagery and National Identity in England and the United States*. Princeton: Princeton University Press.

Daumal, René. 1970/1982. *Rasa or Knowledge of the Self: Essays on Indian Aesthetics and Selected Sanskrit Studies*. Translated by Louise Landes Levi. New York: New Directions Books.

Davidson, Joyce. 2003. *Phobic Geographies: The Phenomenology and Spatiality of Identity*. Aldershot, UK: Ashgate.

Deleuze, Gilles, and Félix Guattari. 1987. *A Thousand Plateaus: Capitalism and Schizophrenia*. Translated by Brian Massumi. Minneapolis: University of Minnesota Press.

Demel, Walter. 2001. "The Images of the Japanese and the Chinese in Early Modern Europe: Physical Characteristics, Customs and Skills. A Comparison of Different Approaches to the Cultures of the Far East." *Itinerario* 25: 34–53.

Derideaux, Pieter. 2006. "Inscription at Ngantang." Nov. 10, 2006. <http://www
.geocities.com/pieterderideaux/inscription.html>.

Dhoraisingam, Samuel. 2006. *Peranakan Indians of Singapore and Malaka: Indian Babas and Nonyas-Chitty Melaka*. Singapore: Institute of Southeast Asian Studies.

Dick, H. 1996. "The Emergence of a National Economy, 1808–1990s." In *Historical Foundations of a National Economy in Indonesia, 1890s–1990s*, edited by J. Lindblad, 21–51. Amsterdam: North Holland.

Djamaris, Edwar. 1984. *Menggali Khazanah Sastra Melayu Klasik (Sastra Indonesia Lama): Sastra Tradisional, Sastra Berisi Sejarah, Sastra Pengaruh Islam*. Jakarta: Proyek Penerbitan Buku Sastra Indonesia.

Douglas, Susan. 2000. "Narcissism as Liberation." In *The Gender and Consumer Culture Reader*, edited by Jennifer Scanlon, 267–282. New York: New York University Press.

Drakeley, Steven. 2005. *The History of Indonesia*. Westport, CT: Greenwood Press.

Dua, J. 2006. "Ramayana Tradition as a Historical Source Material." In *Ramayana Tradition in Historical Perspective*, edited by D. Saklani, 92–109. Delhi, India: Pratibha Prakashan.

Dwipayana, Aagn. 2001. *Kelas dan Kasta: Pergulatan Kelas Menengah Bali*. Yogyakarta: Lapera.

Dyer, Richard. 1997. *White*. New York: Routledge.

Ebo, Bosah. 2001. *Cyberimperialism?: Global Relations in the New Electronic Frontier*. Westport, CT: Praeger.

Ebo, Bosah, ed. 1998. *Cyberghetto or Cybertopia?: Race, Class, and Gender on the Internet*. Westport, CT: Praeger.

Eco, Umberto. 1980. "Function and Sign: The Semiotics of Architecture." In *Signs, Symbols, and Architecture*, edited by Geoffrey Broadbent, Richard Bunt, and Charles Jencks, 11–69. New York: John Wiley and Sons Ltd.

Eliot, Thomas. 1932/1958. *Selected Essays*. London: Faber.

Eliraz, Giora. 2004. *Islam in Indonesia*. Brighton: Sussex.

Enloe, Cynthia. 1989. *Bananas, Beaches, and Bases: Making Feminist Sense of International Politics*. Berkeley: University of California.

Etcoff, Nancy. 1999. *Survival of the Prettiest: The Science of Beauty*. New York: Doubleday.

Fanon, Frantz. 1952/1967. *Black Skin White Masks*. Translated by Charles Markmann. New York: Grove Press.

Farid, Hilmar. 2005. "The Class Question in Indonesian Social Sciences." In *Social Science and Power in Indonesia*, edited by Vedi Hadiz and Daniel Dhakidae, 167–195. Jakarta: Equinox.

Fasseur, C. 1997. "Cornerstone and Stumbling Block: Racial Classification and the Late Colonial State in Indonesia." In *Racial Classification and History*, edited by Nathaniel Gates, 83–108. New York: Garland.

Ferguson, Tamara, and Heidi Eyre. 2000. "Engendering Gender Differences in Shame and Guilt: Stereotypes, Socialization, and Situational Pressures." In *Gender and Emotion: Social Psychological Perspectives*, edited by Agneta H. Fischer, 254–276. Cambridge: Cambridge University Press.

Fields, Jessica. 2005. "'Children Having Children': Race, Innocence, and Sexuality Education." *Social Problems* 52, no. 4: 549–571.

Foucault, Michel. 1977/1979. *Discipline and Punish: The Birth of the Prison*. Translated by Alan Sheridan. New York: Vintage Books.

Foulcher, Keith. 1990. "The Construction of an Indonesian National Culture: Patterns of Hegemony and Resistance." In *State and Civil Society in Indonesia*, edited by Arief Budiman, 301–320. Clayton, Australia: Centre of Southeast Asian Studies.

Foulcher, Keith, and Tony Day, eds. 2002. *Clearing a Space: Postcolonial Readings of Modern Indonesian Literature*. Leiden: KITLV.

Freeman, Carla. 2007. "Neo-liberalism and the Marriage of Reputation and Respectability: Entrepreneurship and the Barbadian Middle Class." In *Love and Globalization: Transformations of Intimacy*, edited by Mark Padilla and Jennifer Hirsch, 3–37. Nashville: Vanderbilt University Press.

Frith, Katherine, ed. 1997. *Undressing the Ad: Reading Culture in Advertising*. New York: Peter Lang.

Geertz, Clifford. 1973. *Interpretation of Cultures*. New York: Basic Books.

———. 1960. *The Religion of Java*. Chicago: University of Chicago Press.

Gilbert, Sandra, and Susan Gubar. 1979. *The Madwoman in the Attic: The Woman Writer and the Nineteenth-Century Literary Imagination*. New Haven, CT: Yale University Press.

Giroux, Henry. 2000. *Stealing Innocence: Youth, Corporate Power, and the Politics of Culture*. New York: St. Martin's Press.

Glenn, Evelyn. 2009. "Consuming Lightness: Modernity, Transnationalism, and Commodification." In *Shades of Difference: Why Skin Color Matters*, edited by Evelyn Glenn, 166–187. Stanford, CA: Stanford University Press.

———. 2008. "Yearning for Lightness: Transnational Circuits in the Marketing and Consumption of Skin Lighteners." *Gender and Society* 22, no. 3: 281–302.

Goffman, Erving. 1979. *Gender Advertisements*. Cambridge, MA: Harvard University Press.

Goldman, Robert. 1992. *Reading Ads Socially*. London: Routledge.

Goldman, Robert, trans. 1984. *The Ramayana of Valmiki*. Vol. 1. Princeton: Princeton University Press.

Gormley, Paul. 2005. *The New-Brutality Film: Race and Affect in Contemporary Hollywood Culture*. Bristol, UK: Intellect.

Gouda, Frances. 1995. *Dutch Culture Overseas: Colonial Practice in the Netherlands Indies 1900–1942*. Amsterdam: Amsterdam University Press.

Grewal, Inderpal. 2005. *Transnational America: Feminisms, Diasporas, Neoliberalisms*. Durham, NC: Duke University Press.

Grossberg, Lawrence. 1992. *We Gotta Get Out of This Place: Popular Conservatism and Postmodern Culture*. New York: Routledge.

Gupta, Akhil. 2003. "The Song of the Nonaligned World: Transnational Identities and the Reinscription of Space in Late Capitalism." In *The Anthropology of Space and*

Place: Locating Culture, edited by Setha M. Low and Denise Lawrence-Zuniga, 321–334. Malden, MA: Blackwell.

Gwin, Minrose. 1996. "Space Travel: The Connective Politics of Feminist Reading." *Signs: Journal of Women in Culture and Society* 21, no. 4: 870–905.

Hadi, Abdul. 2002. "Islam dan Dialog Kebudayaan: Perspektif Hermeneutik." In *Agama dan Pluralitas Budaya Lokal*, edited by Zakiyuddin Baidhawy and Mutohharun Jinan, 113–137. Surakarta, Indonesia: Pusat Studi Budaya dan Perubahan Sosial Universitas Muhammadiyah Surakarta.

Hadiz, Vedi. 2003. "Changing State-Labour Relations." In *Challenging Authoritarianism in Southeast Asia*, edited by Ariel Heryanto and Sumit Mandal, 90–116. London: Routledge.

Haldrup, Michael, Lasse Koefoed, and Kirsten Simonsen. 2008. "Practising Fear: Encountering O/other Bodies." In *Fear: Critical Geopolitics and Everyday Life*, edited by Rachel Pain and Susan Smith, 117–127. Hampshire, UK: Ashgate.

Hall, Dennis. 2006. "Spears' Space: The Play of Innocence and Experience in the Bare-Midriff Fashion." *The Journal of Popular Culture* 39, no. 6: 1025–1034.

Hall, Kenneth. 2005. "Traditions of Knowledge in Old Javanese Literature, c. 1000–1500." *Journal of Southeast Asian Studies* 36, no. 1: 1–27.

Hall, Ronald. 2005. "The Euro-Americanization of Race: Alien Perspective of African Americans vis-à-vis Trivialization of Skin Color." *Journal of Black Studies* 36, no. 1: 116–129.

———. 1995. "The Bleaching Syndrome: African Americans' Response to Cultural Domination Vis-à-Vis Skin Color." *Journal of Black Studies* 26, no. 2: 172–184.

Haraway, Donna. 1988. "Situated Knowledges: The Science Question in Feminism and the Privilege of Partial Perspective." *Feminist Studies* 14, no. 3: 575–599.

Harding, Jennifer, and E. Deidre Pribram. 2009. *Emotions: A Cultural Studies Reader*. London: Routledge.

———. 2004. "Losing Our Cool? Following Williams and Grossberg on Emotions." *Cultural Studies* 18, no. 6: 863–883.

———. 2002. "The Power of Feeling: Locating Emotions in Culture." *European Journal of Cultural Studies* 5, no. 4: 407–426.

Harré, Rom. 1991. *Physical Being: A Theory for a Corporeal Psychology*. Oxford: Blackwell.

Harré, Rom, and Grant Gillett. 1994. *The Discursive Minds*. Thousand Oaks, CA: Sage.

Harré, Rom, and W. Gerrod Parrott. 1996. "Embarrassment and the Threat to Character." In *The Emotions: Social, Cultural and Biological Dimensions*, edited by Rom Harré and W. Gerrod Parrott, 39–56. London: Sage.

Harvey, David. 2009. *Cosmopolitanism and the Geographies of Freedom*. New York: Columbia University Press.

Hatley, Barbara. 1994. "Cultural Expression." In *Indonesia's New Order: The Dynamics of Socio-economic Transformation*, edited by Hal Hill, 216–266. Honolulu: University of Hawai'i Press.

Hellwig, Tineke. 1994. *In the Shadow of Change: Women in Indonesian Literature*. Berkeley: University of California Press.

Hellwig, Tineke, and Eric Tagliacozzo, eds. 2009. *The Indonesia Reader: History, Culture, Politics.* Durham, NC: Duke University Press.

Hemmings, Clare. 2005. "Invoking Affect: Cultural Theory and the Ontological Turn." *Cultural Studies* 19, no. 5: 548–567.

Heryanto, Ariel. 1999. "The Years of Living Luxuriously: Identity Politics of Indonesia's New Rich." In *Culture and Privilege in Capitalist Asia*, edited by Michael Pinches, 159–187. London: Routledge.

Higgins, Kathleen. 2007. "An Alchemy of Emotion: *Rasa* and Aesthetic Breakthroughs." In *Global Theories of the Arts and Aesthetics*, edited by Susan Feagin, 43–54. Malden, MA: Blackwell.

Hintzen, Perry Clude, and Jean M Rahier. 2003. "Introduction: From Structural Politics to the Politics of Deconstruction: Self-Ethnographies Problematizing Blackness." In *Problematizing Blackness: Self-Ethnographies by Black Immigrants to the United States*, edited by Percy C. Hintzen and Jean M. Rahier, 1–20. New York: Routledge.

Hitchcock, Michael, and Victor King. 1997. "Introduction: Malay-Indonesian Identities." In *Images of Malay-Indonesian Identity*, edited by Michael Hitchcock and Victor T. King, 1–17. Kuala Lumpur: Oxford University Press.

Holbert, Steve, and Lisa Rose. 2004. *The Color of Guilt and Innocence: Racial Profiling and Police Practices in America.* San Ramon, CA: Page Marque.

Hoschild, Arlie. 1983. *The Managed Heart: Commercialization of Human Feeling.* Berkeley: University of California Press.

hooks, bell. 2003. *Rock My Soul: Black People and Self-Esteem.* New York: Atria.

Hunter, Margaret. 2005. *Race, Gender, and the Politics of Skin Tone.* New York: Routledge.

Hunter, Thomas. 2002. "Indo as Other: Identity, Anxiety and Ambiguity in 'Salah Asoehan.'" In *Clearing a Space: Postcolonial Readings of Modern Indonesian Literature*, edited by Keith Foulcher and Tony Day, 109–143. Leiden: KITLV.

Inge, Thomas. 2004. "Walt Disney's Snow White: Art, Adaptation, and Ideology." *Journal of Popular Film and Television* 32, no. 3: 132–142.

Ingraham, Chrys. 1999. *White Weddings: Romancing Heterosexuality in Popular Culture.* New York: Routledge.

Irsyam, Tri Wahyuning. 1985. "Golongan Etnis Cina Sebagai Pedagang Perantara di Indonesia (1870–1930)." Jakarta: Depdikbud Direktorat Sejarah dan Nilai Tradisional Inventarisasi dan Dokumen Sejarah Nasional.

Ismail, M. Gade. 1996. "Aceh's Dual Economy during the Late Colonial Period." *Historical Foundations of a National Economy in Indonesia, 1890s–1990s*, edited by J. Lindblad, 229–248. Amsterdam: North Holland.

Jacoby, Mario. 1994/2001. *Shame and the Origins of Self-Esteem: A Jungian Approach*, translated by Douglas Whitcher. New York: Routledge.

Jaggar, Alison. 1989. "Love and Knowledge: Emotion in Feminist Epistemology." In *Gender/Body/Knowledge: Feminist Reconstructions of Being and Knowing*, edited by Alison Jaggar and Susan Bordo, 145–171. New Brunswick, NJ: Rutgers University Press.

Jhally, Sut. 2003. "Image-Based Culture: Advertising and Popular Culture." In *Gender, Race, and Class in Media*, edited by Gail Dines and Jean Humez, 2nd ed., 249–257. Thousand Oaks, CA: Sage.

Kahin, Audrey, and George Kahin. 1995. *Subversion as Foreign Policy: The Secret Eisenhower and Dulles Debacle in Indonesia*. New York: New Press.

Kartajaya, Hermawan. 2004. *Marketing in Venus*. Jakarta: Gramedia.

Kartini. 2002. *Habis Gelap Terbitlah Terang*. Jakarta: Balai Pustaka.

Kartodirdjo, Sartono. 2001. *Indonesian Historiography*. Yogyakarta: Kanisius.

Kasetsiri, Charnvit. 2003. "The Construction of National Heroes and/or Heroines." In *Southeast Asia Over Three Generations*, edited by James T. Siegel and Audrey R. Kahin, 13–25. Ithaca, NY: Southeast Asia Program Publications Cornell University.

Kawashima, Terry. 2002. "Seeing Faces, Making Races: Challenging Visual Tropes of Racial Difference." *Meridians* 3, no. 1: 161–190.

Keeler, Ward. 1983. "Shame and Stage Fright in Java." *Ethos* 11, no. 3: 152–165.

Kim, Nadia. 2008. *Imperial Citizens: Koreans and Race from Seoul to LA*. Stanford, CA: Stanford University Press.

Kinsman, Phil. 1995. "Landscape, Race and National Identity: The Photography of Ingrid Pollard." *Area* 27, no. 4: 300–310.

Kirby, Kathleen. 1993. "Thinking through the Boundary: The Politics of Location, Subjects, and Space." *boundary 2* 20, no. 2: 173–189.

Kirkham, Pat, and Alex Weller. 2003. "Cosmetics: A Clinique Case Study." In *Gender, Race, and Class in Media*, edited by Gail Dines and Jean Humez, 2nd ed., 268–273. Thousand Oaks, CA: Sage.

Knight, G. Roger. 2000. *Narratives of Colonialism: Sugar, Java, and the Dutch*. Huntington, NY: Nova Science Publishers.

Kolko, Beth, Lisa Nakamura, and Gilbert Rodman, eds. 2000. *Race in Cyberspace*. New York: Routledge.

Krishnamoorthy, K. 1986. "The Relevance of Rasa Theory to Modern Literature." In *Some Aspects of The Rasa Theory*, edited by V. Kulkarni, 81–96. Delhi: B.L. Institute of Indology.

Krishnaswamy, Revathi. 1998. *Effeminism: The Economy of Colonial Desire*. Ann Arbor: University of Michigan Press.

Kulkarni, V. M. 1986. "Abhinavagupta on the Alaukika Nature of Rasa." In *Some Aspects of The Rasa Theory*, edited by V. Kulkarni, 28–42. Delhi: B.L. Institute of Indology.

Kurasawa, Aiko. 1990. "'Marilah Kita Bersatu!' Japanese Propaganda in Java 1942–1945." In *Asian Panorama: Essays in Asian History, Past and Present*, edited by K. M. de Silva, Sirima Kiribamune, and C. R. de Silva, 486–497. New Delhi: Vikas.

Kusno, Abidin. 2007. "Space, Power and Identity: Patches of the Postcolonial Past, Present and Future Jakarta." *Journal of Comparative Cultural Studies in Architecture* 1: 37–42.

———.2000. *Behind the Postcolonial: Architecture, Urban Space and Political Cultures in Indonesia*. London: Routledge.

La Botz, Dan. 2001. *Made in Indonesia: Indonesian Workers since Suharto*. Cambridge: South End Press.

Laffan, Michael. 2003. *Islamic Nationhood and Colonial Indonesia*. London: Routledge.

Laurel, Brenda. 1993. *Computer as Theater*. Reading, MA: Addison-Wesley.

Lefebvre, Henri. 1991. *The Production of Space*. Translated by Donald Nicholson-Smith. Oxford: Blackwell.

Lehtinen, Ullalina. 1998. "How Does One Know What Shame Is? Epistemology, Emotions, and Forms of Life in Juxtaposition." *Hypatia* 13, no. 1: 56–77.

Leiliyanti, Eva. 2003. "Konstruksi Identitas Perempuan Dalam Majalah *Cosmopolitan* Indonesia." *Jurnal Perempuan* 28: 69–84.

Leirissa, R. 1994. "'Copracontracten': An Indication of Economic Development in Minahasa during the Late Colonial Period." In *Historical Foundations of a National Economy in Indonesia, 1890s–1990s*, edited by J. Lindblad, 265–277. North Holland: Royal Netherlands Academy of Arts and Sciences.

Leiss, William, Stephen Kline, and Sut Jhally. 1986. *Social Communication in Advertising*. Toronto: Methuen.

Leung, Freedom, Sharon Lam, and Sherrien Sze. 2001. "Cultural Expectations of Thinness in Chinese Women." *Eating Disorders* 9: 339–350.

Liddle, William, R. 1996. *Leadership and Culture in Indonesian Politics*. Sydney: Asian Studies Association of Australia in association with Allen & Unwin.

Lindblad, J. 1994. "Business Strategies in Late Colonial Indonesia." In *Historical Foundations of a National Economy in Indonesia, 1890s–1990s*, edited by J. Lindblad, 207–227. Amsterdam: Royal Netherlands Academy of Arts and Sciences.

Lindquist, Johan. 2009. *The Anxieties of Mobility: Migration and Tourism in the Indonesian Borderlands*. Honolulu: University of Hawai'i Press.

———. 2004. "Veils and Ecstasy: Negotiating Shame in the Indonesian Borderlands." *Ethnos* 69, no. 4: 487–508.

Lindsay-Hartz, Janice Joseph de Rivera, and Michael Mascolo. 1995. "Differentiating Guilt and Shame and Their Effects on Motivation." In *Self-Conscious Emotions: The Psychology of Shame, Guilt, Embarrassment, and Pride*, edited by June Tangney and Kurt Fisher, 274–300. New York: Guilford Press.

Lipsitz, George. 2007. "The Racialization of Space and the Spatialization of Race: Theorizing the Hidden Architecture of Landscape." *Landscape Journal* 26, no. 1: 10–23.

———. 1998/2006. *The Possessive Investment in Whiteness: How White People Profit from Identity Politics*. Philadelphia: Temple University Press.

Locher-Scholten, Elsbeth. 2000. *Women and the Colonial State: Essays on Gender and Modernity in the Netherlands Indies 1900–1942*. Amsterdam: Amsterdam University Press.

———. 1992. "The Nyai in Colonial Deli: A Case of Supposed Mediation." In *Women and Mediation in Indonesia*, edited by Sita van Bemmelen, Madelon Djajadiningrat-Niewenhuis, Elsbeth Locher-Scholten, and Elly Touwen-Bouwsma, 265–280. Leiden: KITLV Press.

————. 1986. "European Images of Japan and Indonesian Nationalism before 1942." In *The Indonesian Revolution*, edited by J. van Goor, 9–33. Utrecht: Instituut voor Geschiedenis.

Lohanda, Mona. 2002. *Growing Pains: The Chinese and the Dutch in Colonial Java, 1890–1942*. Jakarta: Yayasan Cipta Loka Caraka.

Low, Setha, and Denise Lawrence-Zúñiga. 2003. "Locating Culture." In *The Anthropology of Space and Place: Locating Culture*, edited by Setha M. Low and Denise Lawrence-Zúñiga, 1–48. Malden, MA: Blackwell.

Lowe, Lisa. 1996. *Immigrant Acts: On Asian American Cultural Politics*. Durham, NC: Duke University Press.

Lucas, Anton. 1997. "Images of the Indonesian Woman during the Japanese Occupation 1942–45." In *Women Creating Indonesia: The First Fifty Years*, edited by Jean Gelman Taylor, 52–90. Clayton, Australia: Monash Asia Institute.

Lutz, Catherine. 1988. *Unnatural Emotions: Everyday Sentiments on a Micronesian Atoll and Their Challenge to Western Theory*. Chicago: University of Chicago Press.

Macedo, Donald, and Panayota Gounari, eds. 2006. "Globalization and the Unleashing of New Racism: An Introduction." In *The Globalization of Racism*, edited by Donald Macedo and Panayota Gounari, 3–35. Boulder: Paradigm.

Machin, David, and Joanna Thornborrow. 2003. "Branding and Discourse: The Case of *Cosmopolitan*." *Discourse and Society* 14, no. 4: 453–471.

Mackie, J. 1994. "The 1941–1965 Period as an Interlude in the Making of a National Economy: How Should We Interpret It?" In *Historical Foundations of a National Economy in Indonesia, 1890s–1990s*, edited by J. Lindblad, 331–347. Amsterdam: Royal Netherlands Academy of Arts and Sciences.

Mackie, Jamie, and Andrew MacIntyre. 1994. "Politics." In *Indonesia's New Order: The Dynamics of Socio-economic Transformation*, edited by Hal Hill, 1–53. Honolulu: University of Hawai'i Press.

Mackie, Vera. 1995. "Liberation and Light: The Language of Opposition in Imperial Japan." *East Asian History*, no. 9: 99–115.

Malik, Dedy Djamaluddin. 1997. "Media Massa dan Urbanisasi Kesadaran." In *Hegemoni Budaya*, edited by Idi Dubandy Ibrahim and Dedy Djamaluddin Malik, 212–218. Yogyakarta: Bentang.

Malna, Afrizal. 2000. *Sesuatu Indonesia*. Yogyakarta: Bentang.

Mandal, Sumit. 1994. "Finding Their Place: A History of Arabs in Java under Dutch Rule, 1800–1924." PhD diss., Columbia University.

Massumi, Brian. 2002. *Parables for the Virtual: Movement, Affect, Sensation*. Durham, NC: Duke University Press.

McLaren, Peter. 1995. *Critical Pedagogy and Predatory Culture: Oppositional Politics in a Postmodern Era*. London: Routledge.

McMachon, Kathryn. 1990. "The *Cosmopolitan* Ideology and the Management of Desire." *Journal of Sex Research* 27, no. 3: 381–396.

Mercer, Kobena. 1987. "Black Hair/Style Politics." *New Formations* 3: 33–55.

Meyer, Johann. 2003. *Sexual Life in Ancient India: A Study in the Comparative History of Indian Culture.* Vols. 1 and 2. London: Kegan Paul Limited.

Mirpuri, Gouri. 1990. *Indonesia.* New York: Cavendish.

Mirzoeff, Nicholas. 1999. *An Introduction to Visual Culture.* London: Routledge.

Mrázek, Rudolf. 1999. "From Darkness to Light: Optics of Policing in Late-Colonial Netherlands East Indies." In *Figures of Criminality in Indonesia, the Philippines, and Colonial Vietnam,* edited by Vicente Rafael, 13–46. Ithaca, NY: Southeast Asia Program Publications, Cornell University.

Mulkhan, Abdul. 2002. "Muhammadiyah dalam Keragaman Budaya Lokal." In *Agama dan Pluralitas Budaya Lokal,* edited by Zakiyuddin Baidhawy and Mutohharun Jinan, 205–226. Surakarta: Pusat Studi Budaya dan Perubahan Sosial U. Muhammadiyah Surakarta.

Mulyana, Slamet. 2005. *Runtuhnya Kerajaan Hindu-Jawa dan Timbulnya Negara-Negara Islam di Nusantara.* Yogyakarta: LKIS.

———. 1979. *Negarakertagama dan Tafsir Sejarahnya.* Jakarta: Bhratara.

Nakamura, Lisa. 2008. *Digitizing Race: Visual Cultures of the Internet.* Minneapolis: University of Minnesota Press.

———. 2002. *Cybertypes: Race, Ethnicity, and Identity on the Internet.* New York: Routledge.

Nandi, Tapasvi. S. 1986. "Wordly Nature of Rasa." In *Some Aspects of The Rasa Theory,* edited by V. Kulkarni, 43–53. Delhi: B.L. Institute of Indology.

———.1973. *The Origin and Development of the Theory of Rasa and Dhvani in Sanskrit Poetics.* Ahmedabad, India: Gujarat University Theses Publications Series.

Nash, Catherine. 1996. "Reclaiming Vision: Looking at Landscape and the Body." In *Gender, Place and Culture: A Journal of Feminist Geography* 3, no. 2: 149–170.

Nelson, Michelle, and Hye-Jin Paek. 2005. "Cross-Cultural Differences in Sexual Advertising Content in a Transnational Women's Magazine." *Sex Roles* 53, no. 5/6: 371–383.

Noble, Greg, and Scott Poynting. 2008. "Neither Relaxed nor Comfortable: The Affective Regulation of Migrant Belonging in Australia." In *Fear: Critical Geopolitics and Everyday Life,* edited by Rachel Pain and Susan Smith, 129–138. Hampshire, UK: Ashgate.

Omi, Michael, and Howard Winant. 1994. *Racial Formation in the United States: From the 1960s to the 1990s.* New York: Routledge.

Ong, Aihwa. 1999. *Flexible Citizenship: The Cultural Logics of Transnationality.* Durham, NC: Duke University Press.

Onghokham. 1997. "*Show* Kemewahan, Suatu Simbol Sukses." In *Ecstasy Gaya Hidup: Kebudayaan Pop dalam Masyarakat Komoditas Indonesia,* edited by Idi Ibrahim, 175–179. Bandung: Mizan.

O'Reilly, Dougald. *Early Civilizations of Southeast Asia.* Lanham, MD: Altamira, 2007.

Paasonen, Susanna. 2005. *Figures of Fantasy: Internet, Women and Cyberdiscourse.* New York: Peter Lang.

Parameswaran, Radhika, and Kavitha Cardoza. 2009. "Melanin on the Margins: Advertising and the Cultural Politics of Fair/Light/White Beauty in India." *Journalism and Communication Monographs* 11, no. 3: 213–274.

Patankar, R. B. 1986. "Does the Rasa Theory Have Any Modern Relevance?" In *Some Aspects of The Rasa Theory*, edited by V. Kulkarni, 110–120. Delhi: B.L. Institute of Indology.

Pathak, Madhusudan Madhavlal. 1968. *Similes in the Ramayana*. Baroda: The Maharaja Sayajirao University of Baroda.

Pattynama, Pamela. 2007. "Memories of Interracial Contacts and Mixed Race in Dutch Cinema." *Journal of Intercultural Studies* 28, no. 1: 69–82.

Peletz, Michael. 1996. *Reason and Passion: Representations of Gender in a Malay Society*. Berkeley: University of California Press.

Peiss, Kathy. 1998. *Hope in a Jar: The Making of America's Beauty Culture*. New York: Metropolitan.

Phalgunadi, I. 1995. *Indonesian Mahabbharata Bhismaparva*. New Delhi: Pradeep.

Pierre, Jemima. 2008. "'I Like Your Colour!' Skin Bleaching and Geographies of Race in Urban Ghana." *Feminist Review* 90: 9–29.

Pile, Steve. 2009. "Emotions and Affect in Recent Human Geography." *Transactions of the Institute of British Geographers* 35: 5–20.

Porteus, Douglas. 1985. "Smellscape." *Progress in Human Geography* 9: 356–378.

Post, P. 1994. "Characteristics of Japanese Entrepreneurship in the Pre-War Indonesian Economy." In *Historical Foundations of a National Economy in Indonesia, 1890s–1990s*, edited by J. Lindblad, 297–314. Amsterdam: Royal Netherlands Academy of Arts and Sciences.

Prabasmoro, Aquarini. 2003. *Becoming White: Representasi Ras, Kelas, Femininitas dan Globalitas Dalam Iklan Sabun*. Yogyakarta: Jalasutra.

Pred, Allan. 2000. *Even in Sweden: Racisms, Racialized Spaces, and the Popular Geographical Imagination*. Berkeley: University of California Press.

Probyn, Elspeth. 2005. *Blush: Faces of Shame*. Minneapolis: University of Minnesota Press.

———. 2003. "The Spatial Imperative of Subjectivity." In *Handbook of Cultural Geography*, edited by Kay Anderson, Mona Domosh, Steve Pile, and Nigel Thrift, 290–299. London: Sage.

Protschky, Susie. 2008. "The Colonial Table: Food, Culture and Dutch Identity in Colonial Indonesia." *Australian Journal of Politics and History* 54, no. 3: 346–357.

Qurtuby, Sumanto Al. 2003. *Arus Cina-Islam-Jawa: Bongkar Sejarah atas Peranan Tionghoa dalam Penyebaran Agama Islam di Nusantara Abad XV & XVI*. Yogyakarta: Inspeal.

Raben, Remco. 1996. "Batavia and Colombo: The Ethnic and Spatial Order of Two Colonial Cities 1600–1800." PhD diss., Rijksuniversiteit Leiden.

Rafferty, Ellen. 1984. "Languages of the Chinese of Java—An Historical Review." *The Journal of Asian Studies* 43, no. 2: 247–272.

Ram, Kalpana. 2000. "Dancing the Past into Life: The *Rasa, Nrtta,* and *Raga* of Immigrant Existence." *Australian Journal of Anthropology* 11, no. 3: 261–273.

Rand, Erica. 1994. "Lesbian Sightings: Scoping for Dykes in Boucher and *Cosmo.*" *Journal of Homosexuality* 27, no. 1/2: 123–139.

Reddy, William. 2001. *The Navigation of Feeling: A Framework for the History of Emotions.* Cambridge: Cambridge University Press.

Ricklefs, Merle. 2008/2001. *A History of Modern Indonesia since c. 1200.* Stanford, CA: Stanford University Press.

———. 1987. "Indonesian History and Literature." In *Dari Babad dan Hikayat Sampai Sejarah Kritis,* edited by Teuku Ibrahim Alfian, H. J. Koesoemanto, and Dharmono Hardjowidjono, 199–210. Yogyakarta: Gadjah Mada University Press.

Riyanto, Bedjo. 2000. *Iklan Surat Kabar dan Perubahan Masyarakat di Jawa Masa Kolonial (1870–1915).* Yogyakarta: Tarawang.

Robbins, Bruce. 1998. "Comparative Cosmopolitanisms." In *Cosmopolitics: Thinking and Feeling Beyond the Nation,* edited by Peng Cheah and Bruce Robbins, 246–264. Minneapolis: University of Minnesota Press.

Robson, Stuart. 1981. "Java at the Crossroads: Aspects of Javanese Cultural History in the 14th and 15th Centuries." *Bijdragen tot de taal-, land- en volkenkunde* 137, no. 2/3: 259–292.

Rodaway, Paul. 1994. *Sensuous Geographies: Body, Sense and Place.* London: Routledge.

Rondilla, Joanne. 2009. "Filipinos and the Color Complex: Ideal Asian Beauty." In *Shades of Difference: Why Skin Color Matters,* edited by Evelyn Nakano Glenn, 63–80. Stanford, CA: Stanford University Press.

Rondilla, Joanne, and Paul Spickard. 2007. *Is Lighter Better? Skin Tone Discrimination among Asian Americans.* Lanham, MD: Rowman & Littlefield.

Ropi, Ismatu. 2000. *Fragile Nation: Muslims and Christians in Modern Indonesia.* Jakarta: Logos.

Rosaldo, Michelle. 1983. "The Shame of Headhunters and the Autonomy of Self." *Ethos* 2, no. 3: 135–151.

Rosaldo, Renato. 1989. *Culture and Truth: The Remaking of Social Analysis.* Boston: Beacon Press.

Rose, Gillian, Vivian Kinnaird, and Mandy Morris. 1997. "Feminist Geographies of Environment, Nature and Landscape." In *Feminist Geographies: Explorations in Diversity and Difference,* edited by Women and Geography Study Group of the Royal Geographical Society with the Institute of British Geographers, 146–190. Essex, UK: Longman.

Rutherford, Danilyn. 1998. "Trekking To New Guinea." In *Domesticating the Empire: Race, Gender, and Family Life in French and Dutch Colonialism,* edited by Julia Clancy-Smith and Frances Gouda, 255–271. Charlottesville: University Press of Virginia.

Sahay, Sarita, and Niva Piran. 1997. "Skin-Color Preferences and Body Satisfaction among South Asian-Canadian and European-Canadian Female University Students." *The Journal of Social Psychology* 137, no. 2: 161–171.

Santoso, Fattah. 2002. "Agama dan Keragaman Kebudayaan: Perspektif Peradaban Islam." In *Agama dan Pluralitas Budaya Lokal*, edited by Zakiyuddin Baidhawy and Mutohharun Jinan, 45–59. Surakarta: Pusat Studi Budaya dan Perubahan Sosial U. Muhammadiyah Surakarta.

Santoso, Soewito, trans. 1980. *Ramayana Kakawin*. 3 vols. New Delhi: International Academy of Indian Culture.

Saran, Malini, and Vinod C. Khanna. 2004. *The Ramayana in Indonesia*. Delhi: Ravi Dayal Publisher.

Sarkar, Amal. 1987. *A Study on the Ramayanas*. Calcutta: Ridhhi India.

Sarkar, Himansu B. 1983. "The Ramayana in Southeast Asia: A General Survey." In *Asian Variations in Ramayana*, edited by K. R. Srinivasa Iyengar, 206–220. New Delhi: Sahitya Akademi.

———. 1970. *Some Contribution of India to the Ancient Civilisation of Indonesia and Malaysia*. Calcutta: Kamal.

———. 1934. *Indian Influences on the Literature of Java and Bali*. Calcutta: AMS Press Secretary Greater India Society.

Sarker, Sonita, and Esha Niyogi De, eds. 2002. *Trans-Status Subjects: Gender in the Globalization of South and Southeast Asia*. Durham, NC: Duke University Press.

Schein, Louisa. 1999. "Of Cargo and Satellites: Imagined Cosmopolitanism." *Postcolonial Studies* 2: 345–375.

Schivelbusch, Wolfgang. 1995. *Disenchanted Night: The Industrialization of Light in the Nineteenth Century*. Berkeley: University of California Press.

Scholte, Jan Aart. 1995. "The International Construction of Indonesian Nationhood, 1930–1950." In *Imperial Policy and Southeast Asian Nationalism*, edited by Hans Antlöv and Stein Tonnesson, 191–226. Richmond, Surrey, UK: Curzon Press.

Schulte, Henk Nordholt. 1997. "The State on the Skin: Clothes, Shoes, and Neatness in (Colonial) Indonesia." *Asian Studies Review* 21: 19–39.

Schwartz, Susan. 2004. *Rasa: Performing the Divine in India*. New York: Columbia University Press.

Sears, Laurie. 2004. "Mysticism and Islam in Javanese *Ramayana* Tales." In *The Ramayana Revisited*, edited by Mandakranta Bose, 275–292. New York: Oxford University Press.

Secor, Anna. 2007. "Afterword." In *Women, Religion and Space: Global Perspectives on Gender and Faith*, edited by Karen M. Morin and Jeanne Kay Guelke, 148–158. Syracuse: Syracuse University Press.

Sedgwick, Eve. 2003. *Touching Feeling: Affect, Pedagogy, Performativity*. Durham, NC: Duke University Press.

Sedgwick, Eve, and Adam Frank. 1995. *Shame and Its Sisters: A Silvan Tomkins Reader*. Durham, NC: Duke University Press.

Sekarningsih, Ani. 2000. *Namaku Teweraut*. Jakarta: Yayasan Obor.

Sen, Krishna, and Maila Stivens. 1998. *Gender and Power in Affluent Asia*. London: Routledge.

Shahab, Yasmine. 1975. "Masalah Integrasi Minoritas Arab di Jakarta." Thesis, Universitas Indonesia.

Sherrow, Victoria. 2001. *For Appearance' Sake: The Historical Encyclopedia of Good Looks, Beauty, and Grooming.* Westport, CT: Oryx Press.

Shohat, Ella, ed. 1998. *Talking Visions: Multicultural Feminism in a Transnational Age.* Cambridge, MA: MIT Press.

Shohat, Ella, and Robert Stam. 1994. *Unthinking Eurocentrism: Multiculturalism and the Media.* London: Routledge.

Sidel, John. 2006. *Riots, Pogroms, Jihad: Religious Violence in Indonesia.* Ithaca, NY: Cornell University Press.

Siegel, James. 1998. *A New Criminal Type in Jakarta: Counter-Revolution Today.* Durham, NC: Duke University Press.

Skeggs, Beverley. 2000. "Introduction." In *Transformations: Thinking Through Feminism,* edited by Sara Ahmed and Jackie Stacey, 27–32. London: Routledge.

Sneddon, James. 2003. *The Indonesian Language: Its History and Role in Modern Society.* Sydney: University of New South Wales Press Ltd.

Soekiman, Djoko. 2000. *Kebudayaan Indis dan Gaya Hidup Masyarakat Pendukungnya di Jawa (Abad XVIII–Medio Abad XX).* Yogyakarta: Bentang.

Spooner, Catherine. 2001. "*Cosmo*-Gothic: The Double and the Single Woman." *Women: A Cultural Review* 12, no. 3: 292–305.

Stange, Paul. 1984. "The Logic of *Rasa* in Java." *Indonesia* 38: 113–134.

Stearns, Peter, and Carol Stearns. 1985. "Emotionology: Clarifying the History of Emotions and Emotional Standards." *American Historical Review* 90, no. 4: 813–836.

Steinem, Gloria. 1990/2003. "Sex, Lies and Advertising." In *Gender, Race, and Class in Media,* edited by Gail Dines and Jean Humez, 2nd ed., 223–229. Thousand Oaks, CA: Sage.

Stoddard, Lothrop. 1966. *Pasang Naik Kulit Berwarna.* Translated by Panitia Penerbit. Jakarta: Panitia Penerbit.

Stoler, Ann. 2002. *Carnal Knowledge and Imperial Power: Race and the Intimate in Colonial Rule.* Berkeley: University of California Press.

———. 1996. "A Sentimental Education: Native Servants and the Cultivation of European Children in the Netherlands Indies." In *Fantasizing the Feminine in Indonesia,* edited by Laurie J. Sears, 71–91. Durham, NC: Duke University Press.

———. 1995. *Race and the Education of Desire.* Durham, NC: Duke University Press.

———. 1989. "Making Empire Respectable: The Politics of Race and Sexual Morality in 20th Century Colonial Cultures." *American Ethnologist* 16, no. 4: 634–660.

Strassler, Karen. 2008. "Cosmopolitan Visions: Ethnic Chinese and the Photographic Imagining of Indonesia in the Late Colonial and Early Postcolonial Periods." *The Journal of Asian Studies* 67, no. 2: 395–432.

Sunoto, Kapto. 1992. "Ramayana: A Cultural Legacy in Indonesia." In *Ramayana: Its Universal Appeal and Global Role,* edited by Lallan Prasad Vyas, 50–58. Delhi: Har-Anand Publications.

Sunstein, Cass. 2003. *Why Societies Need Dissent*. Cambridge, MA: Harvard University Press.

Suratno, Siti. 2002. "Agama dan Pluralitas Budaya Lokal: Dialektika Pemerkayaan Budaya Islam-Nasional." In *Agama dan Pluralitas Budaya Lokal*, edited by Zakiyuddin Baidhawy and Mutohharun Jinan, 21–33. Surakarta: Pusat Studi Budaya dan Perubahan Sosial U. Muhammadiyah Surakarta.

Suryadinata, Leo. 1981. *Peranakan Chinese Politics in Java, 1917–1942*. Singapore: Singapore University Press.

Suryakusuma, Julia. 2004. *Sex, Power, and Nation: An Anthology of Writings, 1979–2003*. Jakarta: Metafor Publishing.

Sutherland, Heather. 1979. *The Making of a Bureaucratic Elite*. Singapore: Heinemann.

Talbot, Cynthia. 2001. *Precolonial India in Practice: Society, Region, and Identity in Medieval Andhra*. Oxford: Oxford University Press.

Taussig, Michael. 1999. *Defacement, Public Secrecy, and the Labor of the Negative*. Stanford, CA: Stanford University Press.

Taylor, Gabriele. 1985. *Pride, Shame, and Guilt: Emotions of Self-Assessment*. Oxford: Clarendon.

Taylor, Jean. 2003. *Indonesia: Peoples and Histories*. New Haven, CT: Yale University Press.

———. 1992. "Women as Mediators in VOC Batavia." In *Women and Mediation in Indonesia*, edited by Sita van Bemmelen, Madelon Djajadiningrat-Niewenhuis, Elsbeth Locher-Scholten, and Elly Touwen-Bouwsma, 249–263. Leiden: KITLV Press.

Teeuw, A. 1969. *Siwarātrikalpa of Mpu Tanakun. An Old Javanese Poem, Its Indian Source and Balinese Illustrations*. The Hague: M. Nijhoff.

Thapar, Romila. 2002. *History and Beyond*. New Delhi: Oxford University Press.

———. 2000. *Cultural Pasts: Essays in Early Indian History*. New Delhi: Oxford University Press.

Thiong'O, Ngugi Wa. 1986. *Decolonizing the Mind: The Politics of Language in African Literature*. London: James Currey Ltd.

Thrift, Nigel. 2008. *Non-Representational Theory*. London: Routledge.

———. 2004. "Intensities of Feeling: Towards a Spatial Politics of Affect." *Geografiska Annaler* 86 B, no. 1: 57–78.

Thomas, Lynn. 2009. "Skin Lighteners in South Africa: Transnational Entanglements and Technologies of the Self." In *Shades of Difference: Why Skin Color Matters*, edited by Evelyn Glenn, 188–210. Stanford, CA: Stanford University Press.

Titib, I Made. 1998. *Citra Wanita Dalam Kakawin Ramayana (Cermin Masyarakat Hindu Tentang Wanita)*. Surabaya: Paramita.

Toer, Pramoedya Ananta. 1985. *Sang Pemula*. Jakarta: Hasta Mitra.

Tolia-Kelly, Divya. 2007. "Fear in Paradise: The Affective Registers of the English Lake District Landscape Re-visited." *Senses & Society* 2, no. 3: 329–352.

Tomagola, Tamrin. 1990. "The Indonesian Women's Magazine as an Ideological Medium." PhD diss., University of Essex.

Tong, Sebastian. 1999. "Unexpected Convergences: Bakhtin's Novelistic Discourse and Pramoedya Ananta Toer's 'Epic' Novels." *World Literature Today* 73, no. 3: 481–484.

Touwen-Bouwsma, Elly. 1995. "Japanese Minority Policy: The Eurasians on Java and the Dilemma of Ethnic Loyalty." Paper presented at the First Conference of the European Association for South East Asian Studies Shifting Identities in Southeast Asia: Individual, Community and Nation, 1880–1990s. Leiden, June 29–July 1, 1995.

Tuan, Yi-Fu. 1974/1990. *Topophilia: A Study of Environmental Perception, Attitudes, and Values*. New York: Columbia University Press.

———. 1977. *Space and Place: The Perspective of Experience*. Minneapolis: University of Minnesota Press.

van der Veer, Peter. 2002. "Colonial Cosmopolitanism." In *Conceiving Cosmopolitanism: Theory, Context, and Practice*, edited by Steven Vertovec and Robin Cohen, 165–180. New York: Oxford University Press.

van der Veur, Paul. 1969. "Race and Color in Colonial Society: Biographical Sketches by a Eurasian Woman Concerning Pre-World War II Indonesia." *Indonesia* 8: 69–79.

Van Wichelen, Sonja. 2010. *Religion, Politics and Gender in Indonesia: Disputing the Muslim Body*. New York: Routledge.

Vertovec, Steven, and Robin Cohen. 2002. "Introduction: Conceiving Cosmopolitanism." In *Conceiving Cosmopolitanism: Theory, Context, and Practice*, edited by Steven Vertovec and Robin Cohen, 1–22. New York: Oxford University Press.

Vickers, Adrian. 2005. *A History of Modern Indonesia*. Cambridge: Cambridge University Press.

Vlekke, Bernard. 1960. *Nusantara: A History of Indonesia*. Chicago: Quadrangle.

Vyas, Shantikumar. 1967. *India in the Ramayana Age*. Delhi: Atma Ram and Sons.

Wagatsuma, Hiroshi. 1967. "The Social Perception of Skin Color in Japan." *Daedalus* 96, no. 1: 407–443.

Walton, Susan Pratt. 2007. "Aesthetic and Spiritual Correlations in Javanese Gamelan Music." In *Global Theories of the Arts and Aesthetics*, edited by Susan Feagin, 31–41. Malden, MA: Blackwell.

Waskul, Dennis. 2002/2004. "The Naked Self: Body and Self in Televideo Cybersex." In *Readings on Sex, Pornography, and the Internet*, edited by Dennis Waskul, 35–64. New York: Peter Lang.

Wessel, Ingrid. 1994. "State Nationalism in Present Indonesia." In *Nationalism and Ethnicity in Southeast Asia*, edited by Ingrid Wessel, 33–47. Munich: LIT.

White, Hayden. 1987. *The Content of Form: Narrative Discourse and Historical Representation*. Baltimore: John Hopkins University Press.

Wie, Thee Kian. 1996. "Economic Politics in Indonesia during the Period 1950–1965, in particular with Respect to Foreign Investment." In *Historical Foundations of a National Economy in Indonesia, 1890s–1990s*, edited by J. Lindblad, 315–329. Amsterdam: North Holland.

Wieringa, Saskia. 2007. "'If There is No Feeling . . .': The Dilemma between Silence and Coming Out in a Working-Class Butch/Femme Community in Jakarta." In *Love and Globalization: Transformations of Intimacy in the Contemporary World*, edited by Mark Padilla and Jennifer Hirsch, 70–90. Nashville: Vanderbilt University Press.

Williams, John. 1997. "Connotations of Racial Concepts and Color Names." In *Critical Race Theory*, edited by Nathaniel Gates, 231–240. New York: Garland.

Williams, Raymond. 2009. "On Structure of Feeling." In *Emotions: A Cultural Studies Reader*, edited by Jennifer Harding and E. Deidre Pribram, 35–49. London: Routledge.

Williamson, Judith. 1986. "Woman Is an Island: Femininity and Colonization." In *Studies in Entertainment: Critical Approaches to Mass Culture*, edited by Tania Modleski, 99–118. Bloomington: Indiana University Press.

Wilson, Raymond, III. 1983. "Allusion and Implication in John Fowles's 'The Cloud.'" *Studies in Short Fiction* 20, no. 1: 17–22.

Winant, Howard. 2001. *The World Is a Ghetto: Race and Democracy since World War II*. New York: Basic.

———. 1994. *Racial Conditions: Politics, Theory, Comparisons*. Minneapolis: University of Minnesota Press.

Wissinger, Elizabeth. 2007. "Always on Display: Affective Production in the Modeling Industry." In *The Affective Turn: Theorizing the Social*, edited by Patricia Clough with Jean Halley, 231–261. Durham, NC: Duke University Press.

Wolf, Naomi. 1992. *The Beauty Myth: How Images of Beauty Are Used against Women*. New York: Anchor.

Wood, Nichola. 2002. "'Once More with Feeling': Putting Emotion into Geographies of Music." In *Subjectivities, Knowledges, and Feminist Geographies: The Subjects and Ethics of Social Research*, edited by Liz Bondi, 57–71. Lanham, MD: Rowman and Littlefield.

Yeoh, Brenda. 2003, "Postcolonial Geographies of Place and Migration." In *Handbook of Cultural Geography*, edited by Kay Anderson, Mona Domosh, Steve Pile, and Nigel Thrift, 369–380. London: Sage.

Young, Robert. 1995. *Colonial Desire: Hybridity in Theory, Culture and Race*. New York: Routledge.

Yuliati, Dewi, Dhanang Respati Puguh, and Mahendra Pudji Utama. 2002. "Seni Sebagai Media Propaganda Pada Masa Pendudukan Jepang di Jawa (1942–1945): Laporan Penelitian." Semarang: Universitas Diponegoro.

Yusuf, Jumsari. 1984. *Sastra Indonesia Lama Pengaruh Islam*. Jakarta: Pusat Pembinaan dan Pengembangan Bahasa Departemen Pendidikan dan Kebudayaan.

Zane, Kathleen. 1998. "Reflections on a Yellow Eye: Asian I(\Eye/)Cons and Cosmetic Surgery." In *Talking Visions: Multicultural Feminism in a Transnational Age*, edited by Ella Shohat, 161–192. Cambridge, MA: MIT Press.

Zed, Mestika. 1996. "The Dualistic Economy of Palembang in the Late Colonial Period." In *Historical Foundations of a National Economy in Indonesia, 1890s–1990s*, edited by J. Lindblad, 249–264. Amsterdam: North Holland.

Zoetmulder, P. 1974. *Kalangwan: A Survey of Old Javanese Literature*. The Hague: Martinus Nijhoff.

Newspapers and Magazines

Almanak Asia Raya (1943)
Bintang Hindia (1928)
Cosmopolitan (U.S.) June–August 2006–2008
Cosmopolitan (Indonesia) June–August 2006–2008
De Huisvrouw (1938–1939, 1951, 1954–1956)
De Huisvrouw in Deli (1933, 1935)
De Huisvrouw in Indie (1933, 1936–1937, 1940–1941)
De Huisvrouw in Indonesie (1949)
De Huisvrouw in Nord Sumatra (1939–1940)
Djawa Baroe (1943–1945)
Dunia Wanita (1952, 1956–1957)
Femina (1975–1998)
Fu Len (1938)
Keng Po (1933, 1938)
Ketjantikan (1953)
Pantjawarna (1948, 1957–1959)
Pewarta Arab (1933)
Puspa Wanita (1958, 1960)
Soeara Asia (1943–1944)
Suara Perwari (1951, 1953–1955, 1957–1958)
Vereniging van Huisvrouwen Cheribon (1936)
Wanita (1949–1953, 1956–1957)
Warta (1959–1960)

INDEX

States, 58, 97; virtuality, 101–102, 134;
vocabulary in advertisements, 64. *See also*
Caucasians; cosmopolitan whiteness;
Europeans; Indonesian whiteness; skin
color; skin-whitening products
whiteness as beauty ideal: in advertising,
95–96, 104; Caucasian whiteness, 36–37,
50, 51, 84; in contemporary Indonesia,
119–122, 128; in Dutch colonial period,
36–37, 43, 50–53; emotionscape, 72–73,
76–77, 81–82; in Japanese colonial
period, 11, 55–58, 59; Japanese whiteness,
115; in North America, 87, 105–106;
over time, 1; in precolonial period, 10,
15–16, 29–30, 34; resistance, 65; strength,
58–59; transnational circulations, 6, 98,
133, 134–135. *See also* beauty ideals;
Indonesian white beauty
whitening products. *See* skin-whitening
products
Widyawati, 71, 72
Wie, Thee Kian, 66
Williams, John, 58
Williams, Raymond, 22–23

Winant, Howard, 37
Wissinger, Elizabeth, 99, 100
women: Arab, 43; class differences, 52,
57; concubines (*nyais*), 42–43, 46, 117;
control and self-control, 90–91; docile
bodies, 89–90; education, 49; employed,
127; fecundity, 109; femininity, 7, 51,
90, 91; Indo, 42, 43, 65, 72, 78–79, 92;
journalists, 54; as mediators, 42–43; in
modernist Islam, 41; self-confidence,
121–122, 124; solidarity, 121; traditional
clothing, 55–56, 76, 77; work of, 52,
139n11. *See also* beauty ideals; gender

Yardley, 51, 71, 73
yellow skin, 37, 52–53, 65, 68, 76. *See also*
skin color
Yeoh, Brenda, 77
Young, Robert, 34–35

Zane, Kathleen, 84
Zimbabwe, skin-whitening products used in,
6, 84, 109

ABOUT THE AUTHOR

L. Ayu Saraswati is assistant professor of women's studies at the University of Hawaiʻi at Mānoa. She received her Ph.D. in women's studies from the University of Maryland, College Park, and has published in numerous journals including *Feminist Studies*, *Meridians*, and *Feminist Formations*.

OTHER VOLUMES IN THE SERIES

HARD BARGAINING IN SUMATRA: Western Travelers and Toba Bataks in the Marketplace of Souvenirs
  Andrew Causey

PRINT AND POWER: Confucianism, Communism, and Buddhism in the Making of Modern Vietnam
  Shawn Frederick McHale

INVESTING IN MIRACLES: El Shaddai and the Transformation of Popular Catholicism in the Philippines
  Katherine L. Wiegele

TOMS AND *DEES*: Transgender Identity and Female Same-Sex Relationships in Thailand
  Megan J. Sinnott

IN THE NAME OF CIVIL SOCIETY: From Free Election Movements to People Power in the Philippines
  Eva-Lotta E. Hedman

THE TÂY SÂN UPRISING: Society and Rebellion in Eighteenth-Century Vietnam
  George Dutton

SPREADING THE DHAMMA: Writing, Orality, and Textual Transmission in Buddhist Northern Thailand
  Daniel M. Veidlinger

ART AS POLITICS: Re-Crafting Identities, Tourism, and Power in Tana Toraja, Indonesia
  Kathleen M. Adams

CAMBODGE: The Cultivation of a Nation, 1860–1945
  Penny Edwards

HOW TO BEHAVE: Buddhism and Modernity in Colonial Cambodia, 1860–1931
  Anne Ruth Hansen

CULT, CULTURE, AND AUTHORITY: Princess Liễu Hạnh in Vietnamese History
  Olga Dror

KHMER WOMEN ON THE MOVE: Exploring Work and Life in Urban Cambodia
  Annuska Derks

Production Notes for Saraswati | *Seeing Beauty, Sensing Race in Transnational Indonesia*
Cover design by Mardee Melton
Composition by Publishers' Design and Production Services, Inc.
    with display and text type in Garamond Premier Pro
Printing and binding by Sheridan Books, Inc.
Printed on 55 lb. House White Hi-Bulk D37, 360 ppi